P16-35

Focus on Dance IX:

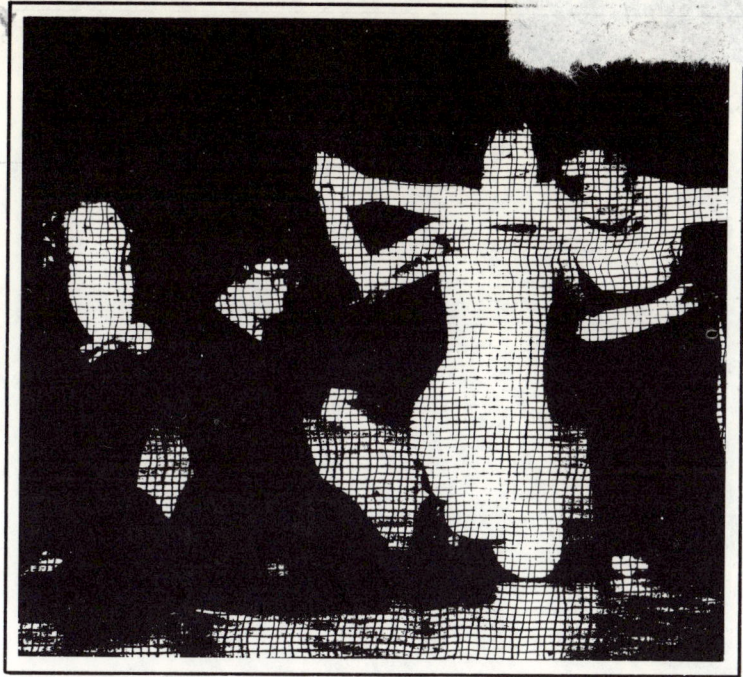

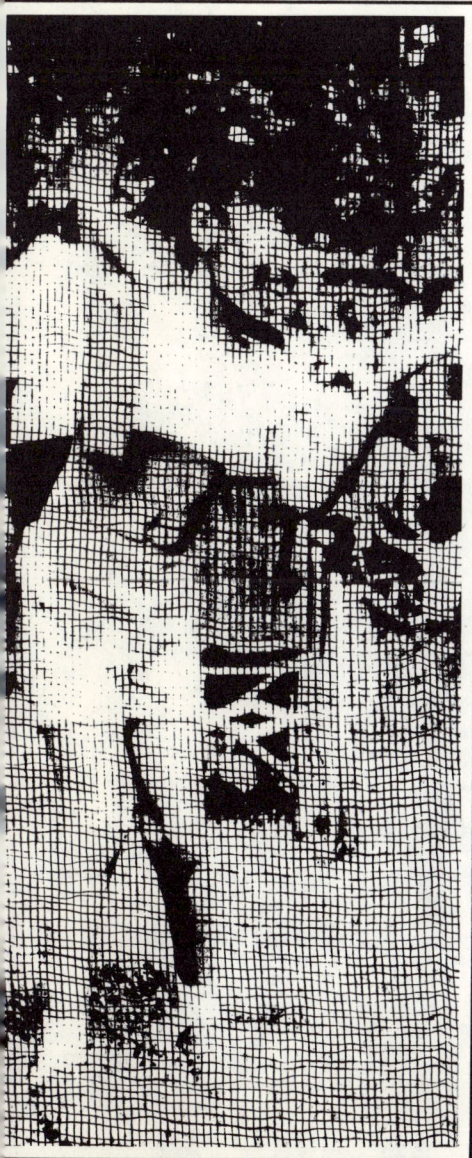

Dance for the Handicapped

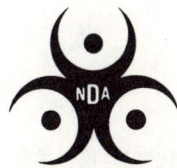

Sponsored by the
NATIONAL DANCE ASSOCIATION
An Association of the American Alliance for Health,
Physical Education, Recreation, and Dance

Foreword

Dance for the handicapped is not new. All over the country, therapists and teachers have been working quietly for years in studios, gymnasia, and other available space. For the most part, these dedicated teachers have been doers, not writers.

Were these teachers to write about their experiences, this volume could expand to many. Time, of course, is the enemy. Teaching dance to the handicapped is a time and energy consuming endeavor. Yet sharing ideas, activities, and methods is as valuable to this field as to any other.

This collection of articles written by people active in the field is intended to initiate a sharing process. Documented in these articles are different approaches, techniques, and philosophies. We made no attempt to present a unified perspective, feeling, after many intense editorial discussions, that the purpose of this monograph was to promote discussion and generate new ideas.

For some readers, certain articles will seem too lengthy and too specific. For others, that specificity may offer the guidance and courage to start a new program. Readers will also note that a number of themes recur throughout the papers: sensory integration, facilitation of expression, fostering positive self concept, and expanding movement repertoires to extend the range of coping behaviors. Perspectives on these themes vary.

As editors, we regret the lack of strong research in dance for the handicapped. The process of careful documentation is, at this time, alien to many people in the field. Again, we are doers, not recorders. Yet we wish to take this opportunity to encourage practitioners to formally document changes in students/clients that result from the dance experience. Such documentaton is needed if dance is to realize its potential as a rehabilitative and actualizing force for persons with handicapping conditions.

Our apologies to the many people in the field whose contributions were not included. Many people working in this area do so quietly and it is only through word of mouth or an occasional publication that one learns about their work.

We sincerely hope this monograph will stimulate interest and sharing and that heretofore untapped resources in the field will enliven future journals.

The editors.
Sally Fitt
Anne Riordan

Contents

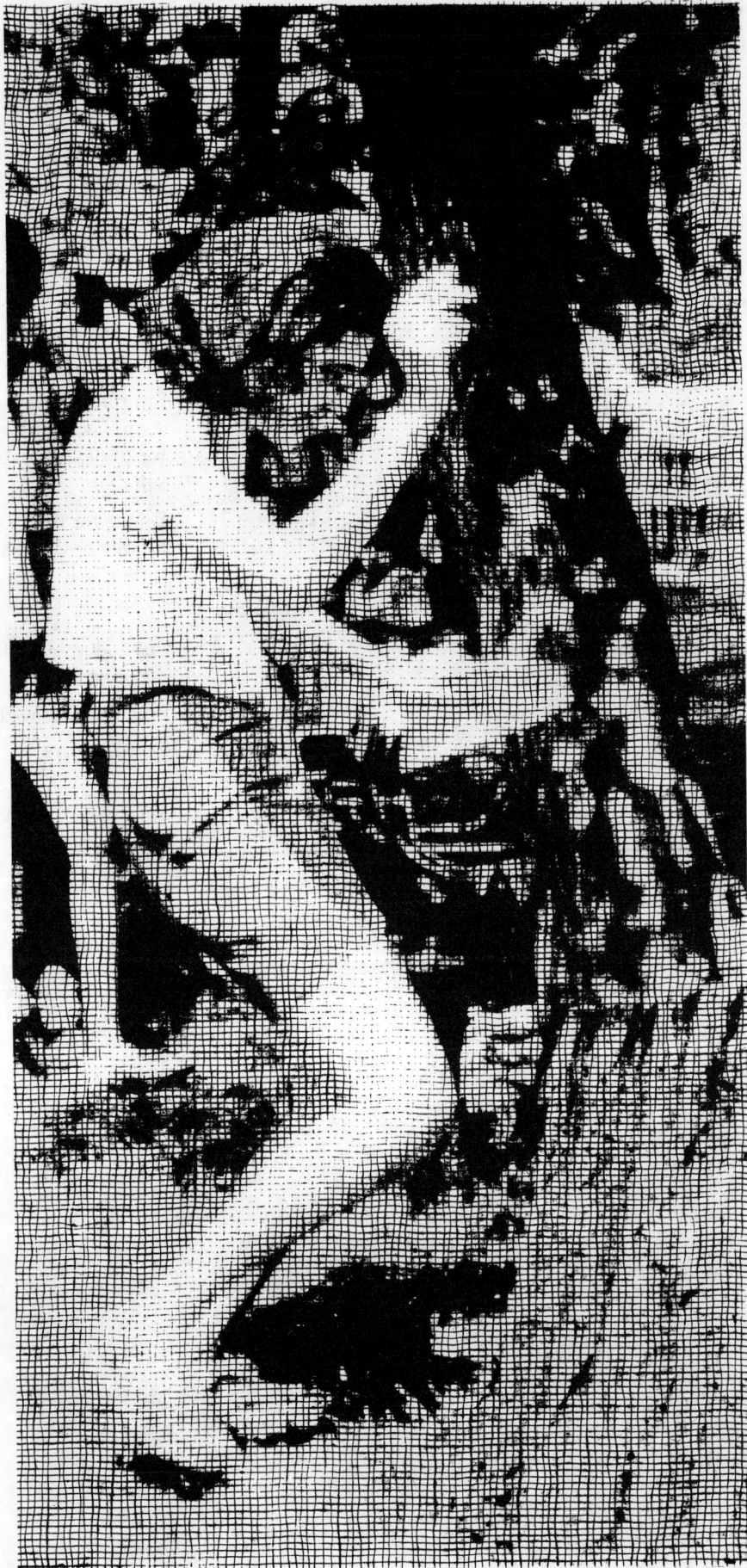

1 Dance for the Handicapped: A Mainstreaming Approach

Cynthia D. Crain

Mainstreaming has been a widely publicized and controversial issue among physical educators for over fifteen years. Although there exists support for proponents of both integration and segregation, the discussion of the mainstreaming concept is quickly shifting from disputation to implementation. This chapter focuses on two concerns primary to mainstreaming in physical education and recreation: (1) generally, the integration of dance activities into recreation and education programs and (2) specifically, the integration of handicapped and non-handicapped persons in the dance program within a physical education and recreation setting.

Public Law 94-142 and the Physical Education and Recreation Program

All parts of the country have been affected by Public Law 94-142 (P.L. 94-142) legislation, as educators and recreators become increasingly aware of the implications this law will have on students, curriculum planning, and evaluation procedures within their programs. Mainstreaming has been decried by some educators; they see it as a punishment for those handicapped persons who are felt to be better off in a segregated program. Others see it as a long awaited vehicle for learning. Whatever the educator's stance, mainstreaming can still be frightening for the unprepared.

Mainstreaming means integrating handicapped children into educational programs. Public Law 94-142 requires that each child be integrated and educated with nonhandicapped children to the maximum degree possible in the least restrictive environment.

The law has not only defined mainstreaming but has further defined the role of the physical education, recreation program (special services) for both handicapped and non-handicapped children and youth. Physical Education is defined by P.L. 94-142 as the development of the following:

1) Physical and motor fitness,
2) Fundamental *motor skills* and *patterns*, and

3) Skills in aquatics, dance, and individual and group games and sports . . . (Stein, 1978: 26).
Therefore, P.L. 94-142 has not only mandated educational programs for the handicapped but has specified *what* developmental learning areas should be covered within the aggregate physical education program. Physical education and recreation, particularly in the areas of games, sports, aquatics, and dance offer opportunities for both handicapped and non-handicapped persons to participate in activities that are educational, recreational, and also therapeutic in nature. Physical education and recreation can contribute to the growth and development of the total person in the psychological, social, and physical domains.

Dance is only one aspect of the aggregate physical education and recreation program, but it is often an area that is misunderstood, abused and misused by practitioners in both fields. While many educators and recreators lack dance knowledge, training, and experience, like other program areas, planned by establishing goals and objectives, and analyzing activities to make use of available method books and records, even the inexperienced or untrained educator can teach a successful dance unit.

The following guideline integrates (1) dance activities in the overall recreation and educational program and (2) handicapped and non-handicapped students in the recreation and physical education program through dance activities.

Integrating a Dance Unit in Physical Education and Recreation

As with any classroom curriculum planning, the physical education teacher instructing a unit on dance must first determine teaching goals, purposes and objectives. Generally, the goal might focus on the students' growth in the social domain through increased awareness of a particular cultural media. The dance unit might expose students to various dance forms, steps, and terminology with one objective to teach a creative dance.

Establishing goals, purposes and objectives probably presents only minor problems for the classroom geared toward non-handicapped students. Yet one might ask how may these be fulfilled in a mainstreaming situation. One most review the goals, purposes and objectives, then reassess and individualize.

The general goal lends itself to both handicapped and nonhandicapped students with relative ease. Let's analyze the objective — teaching a creative dance to students — to a class that has been mainstreamed.

Teaching Dance to Non-Handicapped and Handicapped Persons

Incorporating an idea or theme, within movement is a "tricky" experience for the novice dance teacher; however, the teacher can follow certain guidelines: (1) analyze students' movement ability and repertoire; (2) prepare students for the lesson core to be presented; (3) use teaching aids, equipment, and props when appropriate; (4) adapt and modify the presentation in order to individualize.

Analyzing the movement ability of class members enables the teacher to spot students who will have difficulty moving certain body areas and parts throughout the dance unit. A simplified movement checklist (see Figure 1) guides observation and analysis of movement limitations and enables the teacher to structure the dance activity so that each child will benefit. For example:

> Johnny is a student who was observed to have limited mobility from the waist up. Although Johnny can move his head, arms, and upper torso independently of one another, total coordination and involvement of upper parts simultaneously is slow and difficult.

Once Johnny's limitation has been observed and noted on the checklist, the teacher can stress movement which develops strength and emphasizes muscular integration in this body area when Johnny and the other class members are dancing.

Analyzing the movement repertoire (see Figure 2) provides information concerning each student's (1) dance vocabulary and (2) degree of dance proficiency. The instructor should have each child explain and/or demonstrate the movement components in Figure 2. Lack of knowledge or poor performance should be noted by a check in the *unskilled* column, and excellent performance noted by a check in the *skilled* column. This information identifies students who are familiar with and competent in executing certain dance skills. It also serves to recognize students who lack or are incompetent in these skills. Once the teacher knows the extent of each student's dance knowledge and ability, the

Figure 1. Movement Checklist

I. Body Part Identification	Occurrence	Non-Occurrence
A. Appendages		
arms		
elbows		
legs		
knees		
hands		
feet		
fingers		
toes		
B. Head		
eyebrows		
ears		
mouth		
cheeks		
eyes		
forehead		
chin		
C. Upper Torso		
shoulders		
stomach		
back		
shoulder blades		
neck		
ribs		
D. Lower Torso		
pelvis		
seat		
hips		
waist		
thighs		
E. Combined (for example)		
1. Upper torso		
arms		
head		
waist		
2. Upper/lower torso		
arms		
legs		

second step is to prepare students for the lesson core: learning a creative dance.

Ideally, before presenting a lesson on creative dance, the teacher reeducates or educates students in basic dance skills. The jump, hop, run, skip, and swing are fundamental to *all* dance forms. Additional performing skills inherent in all movement are called "movement components" and "movement qualities." These are *most* important in a mainstreamed dance class, since they provide the teacher with the tools for successful individualization among handicapped and nonhandicapped students.

Movement components include:
1. focus—direction of eyes
2. direction—forward, backward, sideward
3. level/shape/space—high level, fat shape, general space, personal space
4. dynamics—amount of energy exerted in movement
5. tempo—how fast or slow

Movement qualities include:
1. vibratory—rapid shaking of any body part
2. suspension—apex of a jump before descending to earth
3. collapse—falling to the ground
4. sustained—gentle movement with even energy flow
5. swinging—pendulum or arc-like movement
6. percussive — successive sharp movements

Once movement fundamentals have been explored and/or experienced, the teacher may proceed to the third step in teaching a creative dance.

Teaching Aids, Equipment, and Props

Recommended for the educator with limited background in dance, educational records, films, and slide presentations on teaching methodology facilitate teaching. Records for handicapped and nonhandicapped student populations, films, and slide presentations can be offered simultaneously to handicapped and nonhandicapped individuals with little or no modification.

Equipment and props are excellent aids for teaching dance in a mainstreaming situation. Balls can be used for rhythmic exercises; shakers, drums, and tambourines can accompany the creative dance; and scarves which extend the arm illustrate movement qualities while stimulating student enthusiasm for the creative dance performance. Most importantly, equipment, props and aids can (1) serve as a teacher resource, (2) stimulate student interest, (3) facilitate teaching the dance unit in a mainstreaming situation, (4) promote individualization (especially with wheelchair and nonwheelchair persons), and (5) create an edifying learning experience that is also relaxed and fun.

Figure 2. Movement Repertoire Assessment

Rudimentary of Movement	Mechanics Unskilled	Skilled
is able to bend the knees on command	_____	_____
is able to rise on the toes on command	_____	_____
bend the upper body	_____	_____
bend the lower body	_____	_____
lift	_____	_____
grasp	_____	_____
pull	_____	_____
push	_____	_____
over	_____	_____
under	_____	_____
around	_____	_____
inside	_____	_____
outside	_____	_____
beside	_____	_____

Locomotion

	Unskilled	Skilled
walk	_____	_____
run	_____	_____
jump	_____	_____
hop	_____	_____
leap	_____	_____
gallop	_____	_____
slide	_____	_____
skip	_____	_____

Nonlocomotion

	Unskilled	Skilled
collapse	_____	_____
sustain (hold a pose)	_____	_____
swing	_____	_____
bend	_____	_____
turns (in place)	_____	_____
twisting	_____	_____
stamping	_____	_____
clapping	_____	_____

*Directional information as it relates to shape, space and other objects

Individualization within the Dance Unit

When the teacher no longer needs to depend on records and films to determine class content, the final, and perhaps most creative step is to help students express themselves nonverbally through dance. Through dance, students can experience, express, and analyze the process of popping corn. Students and teacher first discuss the sequence of popping corn from pouring oil in the pan, to the heat's expanding the kernels, to the completion when all movement and noise has ceased. Then they can discuss movement components and qualities which best illustrate the popping process. Finally, teacher and students recognize each individual's interpretation of the popping process with regard to abilities, skills, and limitations. Although a wheelchair student without leg mobility will not be able to jump up and down on the floor the student will probably have enough arm strength to isolate the jumping movement in the seat and upper trunk, using the arms in resistance to the wheelchair arm and lifting the body up and down. Individuals adapt and modify the creative dance theme to fit their abilities. With a structurally flexible unit, dance can create an integrated classroom regardless of students' prior skills and dance training.

Conclusion

The key to mainstreaming the handicapped is in the term "least restrictive environment," an integrated environment which can best facilitate learning and growth of handicapped persons. As a "least restrictive environment" dance allows for individualization and physical, and creative activity and expression. Dance can be used in the gym, regular classroom, outdoors, and in school corridors, if necessary. Only the limitations of each individual's imagination circumscribe dance activities.

P.L. 94-142 stipulates the active integration of dance in the education and recreation curricula as a mainstreaming approach for handicapped and nonhandicapped persons. Dance as movement and active participation can be expressed by crippled and wheelchair bound persons, as well as the professionally trained dancer. Not an esoteric field, dance allows all persons to participate in verbal and nonverbal expression and communication through a structured nonrestrictive environment that is challenging, stimulating, and rewarding for all.

References

Lloyd, Marcla L., "The Handicapped Can Dance Too!" *Journal of Physical Education and Recreation*, 49:5, (1978) pp. 52-53.

McGinnis, Rozanne W., "Dance as a Therapeutic Process" *Therapeutic Recreation Journal*, VIII: 4, (1974) pp. 181-186.

Stein, Julian U., "New Laws Open the Field to the Handicapped" *AHICUS*, National Center for Law and the Handicapped, (1978) 3:13.

Tipple, Blanch, "Dance Therapy and Education Program" *Leisurability*, 2:4, (1975) pp. 9-13.

2 The Science of the Art of Giving Directions

Madeline Hunter

"They simply cannot follow directions," is to education what the common cold is to medicine. Everyone complains about it. Every classroom has a problem with it. It's seldom fatal, but the time, energy, and productivity, lost from it is astronomical. Science has not yet solved the problem of the common cold. A scientific attack on students' following directions, however, will go far towards curing that malady. As we study the etiology of *not* following directions, we find there are three causes.

1. *The student does not intend to follow directions.* The direction, "Go directly to your play area," which is followed by the student detouring to enjoy a water fight in the lavatory is an example of a student choosing not to follow directions which clearly he understands and could follow if he wished.

2. *The student is incapable of following the direction.* "Don't be nervous when you stand up to speak," is a typical example. Not so obvious but equally illustrative are the countless directions and school assignments given to students who do not command skills necessary to accomplish them. No matter how hard they try, they cannot follow such directions.

3. *The directions themselves, or the method of giving them are inherently confusing or unclear.* An income tax form is an example with which most persons are only too familiar. Unfortunately, countless directions which generate predictable confusion are given daily in schools.

Of the three reasons for failure to follow directions, the second and third require teachers to apply what is known about learning to follow directions. While one first reason clearly requires a change in the learner so he intends to follow the directions, this too can be accomplished when a sophisticated teacher applies learning "know-how."

Many times the teacher should not be giving directions; the learner should be directing his own behavior. At other times, giving directions facili-

Editors Note: This article was originally written for teachers of the non-handicapped. Yet the information is certainly pertinent for teachers of the handicapped and, therefore, is included in this monograph. It is reprinted from the author's *Prescription for Improved Instruction*, published by Tip Publications, 1976.

tates learning and teaches the skill of "following directions" needed throughout the student's life. "When all else fails, follow the directions," is an admonition that unfortunately is often appropriate.

This chapter focuses on the third reason: the inherent success or failure of the way the directions themselves are given. The reader, however, must always consider: (1) is the student really trying to follow the directions? and (2) is the student able to follow them?

Giving directions involves two steps.

1. Planning—thinking through the directions to determine:

   How many different things must the student remember to do?

   Which of these has he/she done before and which are new to him?

   Can he/she do the new things if he tries?

   How many directions must be given at one time?

   When is the best time to give these directions?

   What is the best sequence for directions that must be given at the same time?

   Should the directions be written or verbal?

   Out of these considerations an operational plan evolves.

2. Giving directions to an individual or a group involves:

   getting attention.

   giving the directions in a way that reflects conscious planning.

   checking understanding.

   modeling behavior.

   translating into action.

   redirecting if necessary.

Successful direction-giving synthesizes elements, but success requires analyzing each separately. Analysis makes it possible to pinpoint an error and remediate it to promote success. In short, science enables us to learn systematically at a conscious level (rather than by blind imitation) how to give directions. If directions are not followed, we can identify what went wrong and adjust.

Planning

It is essential that we break complex behavior into parts. Getting ready for recess involves disposing of finished and/or unfinished work, clearing desks and tables, putting away supplies, being at the appropriate place to be excused, putting on wraps, and knowing where to go when excused. Eventually "get ready for recess," should trigger all these behaviors, but only if each element has previously been learned, which means it *has been taught*. In the same way, "go to the library," "read the chapter and answer the questions", "pass in your papers," and "come to the discussion circle," are composites of simpler directions, each of which must be learned.

How Many Directions?

Do not give more than three directions at the same time is a simple rule of thumb. If the behavior required by any one direction is new or not well learned, that direction should be given alone or paired with a well learned behavior. Seldom (if ever) should directions for two new behaviors be given at the same time. Often complex behaviors can be divided into several sets of directions with one set being accomplished before the next is given. If more than three directions must be given, these should be written or presented in a picture graph for easy student reference.

Timing and Sequence

Deciding *at a conscious level* when each direction should be given can contribute immeasurably to success. Delaying directions for an activity until just before that activity is to be performed causes a great deal of forgetting and confusion. The time to give directions for what to do when you come into the room *tomorrow* morning is not *this* morning. Tomorrow's directions should be given just before dismissal today, or, better, tomorrow morning. This assumes, of course, that following directions, rather than assuming responsibility for remembering over a period of time, is the major objective. The latter also is an important objective, but teaching to *remember* is different.

An example of ending a sequence of directions with the direction to be followed immediately is "after recess today we will go to the auditorium instead of coming back to our room; now check your papers to see if you wish to turn them in or keep them, and excuse yourself for recess as soon as you're ready." Such a set of directions implies the learners have had the experience of going directly to the auditorium and know what to do when they get

there. They know what criteria determine whether papers are finished, and they have had experience excusing themselves. If any one of these is a new behavior, beware — catastrophe is imminent!

Individualizing

Even in direction-giving, individualized instruction is essential for those for whom the direction is too difficult to be accomplished independently. Anticipating these situations allows a teacher to give *dignified* help to such students. "Let's see, Bill, do you want to keep your paper? how many have you finished? do you have more to do? then where will you put your paper?" enables a student who could not function independently to follow directions successfully.

Interestingly, we are aware that some students need extra assistance in reading, writing, and math, but we do not offer them that same support in following directions, no matter how vividly they indicate their need. "If they would only *listen!*" is our panacea.

Written or Oral?

Whether directions should be written or oral is determined by the students' need to "read and do" Both are important skills, but well-planned written directions often provide more practice for the student who must read, comprehend, and transform understanding into performance. Written directions avoid repetition and questions by providing a reference. Even young children can follow picture directions. A lunch sack, a door, and closed lips signify get your lunch and wait quietly at the door. Vivid pictures are often more effective than an adult's voice which many have learned to ignore. Thinking through directions in advance enables us to determine how many should be given at one time, which may be difficult or impossible for some students, what order to use to give directions, and whether they should be written or oral.

Automating

At this point the reader may exclaim, "With all the direction I have to give every day, who has time for all this thinking through?" The answer is "Nobody," but practicing thinking through directions trains one until direction-giving becomes an automatic skill in the same way that practicing driving skills soon makes them automatic.

Giving the Directions

To follow directions, one must understand them. Consequently, the first step of direction-giving is to gain the attention of those who must receive the message. Teachers need to deliberately and systematically develop some method which helps *all* the learners for whom the directions are intended to focus on the source of information. Failure often results when the teacher gives directions when only half of the group is listening or looking.

Giving Directions as Planned

The teacher who gives planned directions reaps the reward. The children will put their lunches away and *then* hang up their wraps, rather than wrestling with jackets, trying to hang on to lunches or having them trampled by other children in the same fix. Children will have heard or be able to read what to do when they enter the room rather than lose precious time in confusion.

Checking Understanding

Unfortunately, giving directions well does not *guarantee* understanding. To ensure that directions will be followed, the teacher must check understanding. "Think of what you will do first. If you know, raise your hand." Then the teacher must *wait*, nudging with her eyes those students who have no intention of "putting their minds in gear." Such teaching clarifies that students are accountable for listening and indicates to the teacher those who don't know what to do. If only a few hands go up, the teacher can observe that directions must be regiven by either children or teacher. If most hands are up, the teacher can decide whether those who don't know can be told by other children or need teacher attention. When the entire set of directions must be checked, the teacher knows that there may have been too many directions.

Modeling the Behavior

Recent brain research, corroborating classroom experience, indicates some students learn easier by hearing, some by reading, and some by seeing. Whenever possible, we provide for the latter group by having a child model the behavior. This also corrects possible misunderstanding. "John, show us what you will do first." "Mary, pretend you have finished; show us where you will put your paper." "Tom, show us where you will get your materials." "Jane, if you need help show us what you will do."

Modeling is effective for others only when it has conscious attention. "Let's watch John and decide if he is following directions. Thumbs up if you think he is." Insist that each student make a judgment. Above all avoid the error of "Sally, did John follow directions?" Saying "Sally" signals the group that no one else will have to think.

Translating into Action

When directions have been given, comprehension checked, and behavior modeled, the teacher must decide if all children or a few at a time will proceed. "If you know what to do you may start; if you're not sure, stay with me (or raise your hand) and I will help you." This strategy will not delay those who are ready but will build in help for those who need it.

The teacher needs to consider whether the total class can get their books, wraps, and lunches, at the same time. Usually "pile ups" can be avoided by releasing a few children while the rest are appropriately engaged, *not* just sitting and waiting. "Be deciding on what you are going to write about (or color, or choose) and I'll ask you to tell me as I excuse you," starts students toward purposeful action while they are waiting.

Remediating

Even with the best directions, occasionally a child doesn't follow. If there are many such children, the directions either have been inappropriate or poorly given. After releasing children to follow directions, the teacher must take a few minutes to check who is following them and who isn't, just as we check arithmetic papers to see who can do the problems and who can't. In the same way we find out who needs help with directions and why. "Bill, what do you need to do first? Where would you go to get it? Show me," helps the uncertain child to learn what to do. *Merely giving the same directions again repeats a teaching action evidence shows did not work.*

The Science of Giving Directions

What is needed for a good set of directions?

Planning. Think through the directions. Decide how many are needed at one time. Determine the order and whether they will be written or oral. Anticipate which students will need help.

Implementation. Get the students' attention, give directions, check comprehension, and model behavior. Release students so they can efficiently perform them. Check to see who needs help and give it in a way that facilitates learning.

The Art of Giving Directions

Once one understands the science of giving directions, that knowledge becomes the launching pad for teaching artistry. The vividness and interest of the directions, the decision of which child needs the experience or status of modeling for the class, the degree to which students become their own direction-givers, the quality and value of the learning task for which directions are given—these are the hallmarks of the teaching artist. We can put the science of direction-giving on paper; the artistry must be your own.

3 Developing Creative Movement Experiences for the Handicapped

Nancy Brooks Schmitz

A child talks animatedly to an adult I assume to be her teacher. Of the three other children with her, one is in a wheelchair. Another blond haired girl appears about seven or eight years old. They are waiting for our program to begin. I noticed them because they arrived early and sat back away from our performing area.

Other children with name tags arrive to fill the four-sided performing area. Quickly involved, I seat children according to the color of their tag. As I introduce myself and my group, the Magic Movers, I try to identify children who might need special help in our program. Again I see the child. Her face is eager. She wears no name tag. As close as I can guess, she is in her early teens. The other children are fifth graders.

"Have you ever told someone a story, or written a poem, or drawn a picture? The Magic Movers sometimes tell stories through movements and mime." With these words our program and movement starts. Our program encourages movement responses from children as we stress communication through movement using the beautiful myths of the Navaho people.

When we reach the point in our program where the children are invited to create environments such as rain forests, deserts, mountains, or seashores, I look for volunteers. Only two hands rise immediately. One is a boy on my right. Not at all reluctant to volunteer, he seems self-confident. The child I was first drawn to also volunteers. As I turn to invite her I see the teacher shaking her head. I wonder if she is communicating that this child is not to join. I invite the child anyway, placing myself close to her if she needs my help. She joins the group she is to work with, and they create a waterfall and a rainforest. As she returns to her seat, in halting speech she says, "I helped!" As the program continues all children have the opportunity to create with their bodies a floor, an abstracted game of "scissors, rock and paper," water monsters, and at last an entire story "How Small Duck Saved the World."

She volunteers many more times, and each time she is selected she listens, watches, and moves according to directions. Each time she shows such joy in doing and being that I find myself caught up in her joy. As the program ends, several children ask questions. One asks "Will you return next year?" "We will if we are asked," I respond. "Did you enjoy the program and movement?" I ask. "Yes," they all answer. As the children return to their classes they come to me or other "Magic Movers" and thank us. She comes up to me, haltingly thanks me, and says she wants to help again next year. "Thank you for moving with us today," I answer. She smiles and leaves, animatedly talking with her teacher about moving and helping. My thoughts during the rest of that tour often return to her joy.

I do not know this child's name. Her story is similar to other children's we have seen all over in our tours. Why aren't the handicapped really included in special arts activities? Although this child and other handicapped children often attend as spectators, all could be participants. They are further handicapped by being placed in the back, away from the activity.

During one performance I moved our props and dancers nearer to a group of physically handicapped children sitting far against a side wall in the gym. Why, by virtue of their handicap, should these children be denied an opportunity to respond to the joy of movement any way they can? Administrators rarely tell us when handicapped children will be present. It appears that schools want to make sure that "normal" children get first chance. Perhaps administrators feel that professional performers are not interested in working with handicapped children. Yet it is possible that dealing with these children's needs is so new that many administrators forget to include them. Since our programs are designed for groups of sixty to eighty children, adding the handicapped group exceeds the quota and the administration designates them "spectators."

It took "Magic Movers" one touring season to realize that if we were interested in involving ourselves with the handicapped, we must inform prospective sponsors that we both welcome the handicapped children's participation in our regular programs and provide special programs and workshops for more severely handicapped children. Through this effort we demonstrate our concern responsibility as artists for segments of communities we visit.

Each child is special and has unique gifts and needs. Handicapped children are no different. Like all children they need to be loved and accepted, to be caught up in the sensuous joy of moving, to develop attention, coordination, and fitness. Handicapped children need to share social and emotional experiences with peers, to feel challenge and success, to create and share creations, to communicate.

Goals and curriculum guides specify that special education ". . . must encompass all functional skills, including behavioral, self-care, gross, and fine motor, nonverbal and verbal communication, safety and health, social and recreational, and functional academic skills." (Bender and Valletutti, 1976) While the arts are not specifically mentioned, incorporating them in the curriculum is justified by "gross and fine motor, nonverbal communication, and . . . social and recreational skills . . . development."

When we limit the handicapped child's involvement with the arts, we limit potential. We also deny opportunities other children take for granted. We tend to think only the average or gifted child will benefit from artistic performances, becoming an informed audience member, arts advocate, or even an artist. We tend also to think of training the average or talented child in the arts. Arts education and specifically dance education, however equally benefit the handicapped and the average child. (Bender and Valletutti, 1976).

Congress has mandated access to all benefits of American society through the removal of physical and program barriers. During committee deliberation of the bill which became P.L. 94-142, the arts were discussed. The Senate report summarized:

> The use of the arts as a teaching tool for the handicapped has long been recognized as a viable, effective way, not only of teaching special skills, but also of reaching youngsters who had otherwise been unreachable. The Committee envisions that programs under this bill could well include an arts component and, indeed, urges that local educational agencies include the arts in programs for the handicapped under this Act. Such a program could cover both appreciation of the arts by the handicapped youngsters and the utilization of the arts as a teaching tool, per se. (U.S. Senate Report 94-169).

Dance/creative movement education can provide opportunities for children to realize their potential by enhancing development of a positive self image, by appealing to the innate need to move, by increasing a child's ability to think creatively through problem-solving, by nurturing positive social interactions, by providing experiences which explore and develop physical and kinesthetic abilities, and by fostering aesthetic experiences.

My interest in teaching persons with handicapping conditions began while I was still in my teens. The local association for the mentally retarded asked me to teach ballet to three eight-year old girls classified as "trainable." One of the girls, Christy, remained my student for six years. The initial goal at that time was to improve the girls' physical coordination, but as I began to work I learned to throw away preconceived ideas about class content and structure. We began to explore new areas of movement and sound. As coordination and self-concept increased, so too did their language, social interactions, and willingness to try new ideas. I began to see that certain teaching methods were more successful than others, and most successful of all were those in which the girls worked with spontaneous movement rather than with specific movement skills. As I became more adept at identifying their strengths, weaknesses, and interests, their progress improved, and they began to share their experience through performance with peers at school. These explorations taught me that handicapped children are sensitive to art experiences both as participants and as audience members. Additionally, I discovered that physical skill has little to do with a successful growth experience. Developing kinesthetic sensibilities and the exhilaration of creation became more important.

The success of my work with this group led me to focus upon four areas of concern within the lesson structure:
1) determining overall objectives;
2) developing opening and closing rituals;
3) developing use of props (textural, visual or aural);
4) discovering diverse ways to communicate our experiences.

As my work progressed, the development of objectives both for the group and for individuals became more important. Establishing objectives requires understanding the developmental level and the particular emotional patterns of each member. Sensitivity to students provides an insight into their developmental needs and problems. Once individual objectives are established, commonalities probably will be discovered among the group. These, plus content objectives, determine the goals.

Suppose we determined that a particular group needed to develop (1) social interaction, (2) an understanding of body parts and their function, and (3) ability to replicate. Some individual members might need to control extraneous physical motion and to learn cooperation.

Early lessons might include follow-the-leader experiences or directives such as "lift your arms way up, wiggle your fingers, slowly bring your arms down," and so on. Lesson objectives might include: exploring movement possibilities with hands, arms, heads, feet, legs, torso; reinforcing concepts of body parts; stressing following directions; developing a sense of duration; developing small and large muscle coordination. Successive lessons might develop social cooperation through partner work (another child, teacher, or aide), using body parts to touch specific places on the partner's body; shaping particular body parts on partner, (shaping partner's hands and arms then placing own hands and arms in same shape), or mirroring each other's movements.

The second concern in the lesson is developing opening and closing rituals. Rituals help students develop a sense of security. If certain patterns are established and maintained, the student has a secure base to leave and to return to when trying new activities. Rituals not only become an eagerly anticipated "old friend," but also reinforce important objectives. An opening ritual might include the use of a musical instrument or a special record to collect the students in a circle or direct them to specific places in the classroom distinctly marked with masking tape or carpet squares). Chanting rhymes with repetitive movements is another way to establish an opening or closing ritual. Relaxation rituals work well for closings, permitting the teacher to quietly encourage and praise each student or to reinforce relaxation. Rituals for taking off and putting on shoes sometimes help to develop continuity from lesson start to finish.

The third concern is including textural, visual or aural props to sensually motivate movement and creativity.

The child's handicap affects the props and movement experiences which the teacher can present. Working with multiply handicapped children, one must provide movement problems in which all children can participate. Sightless children might best be motivated through textural or aural experiences, simple shaping, and directional experiences. Children with hearing losses might benefit from observing demonstrations and using props. The use of props such as scarves, elastics, stretch bags, balloons, ribbons, streamers, or a parachute, will help enhance the quality of the experience for all children. The props provide an interest focus, allowing reluctant children to become involved without exposing themselves. Additionally they provide a means for children to transfer new kinesthetic experiences to their own movement vocabulary while learning basic concepts and building verbal vocabulary. Research concludes:

> Active mastery of a word requires first of all establishment of a "speech foundation" — that is, the gnostic foundation of the word — and secondly, the ability to master visual representation of objects on the one hand and to interact actively with objects on the other. Therefore, we assume that methods to induce speech formation (and first of all the naming of objects) in children with speech pathology should begin with methods to form visual memory, perception, and represent their exactness, specificity, and mobility. Therefore, training should begin with a nonverbal approach using nonverbal material (Tsvetkova and Kuznetsova, 1977).

Other props or aids also provide similar benefits. Mounted pictures of shapes, environments, animals, small toys, simple machines, textures, flannel board characters, clay or pipe cleaners to shape, and instruments to play, explore, all provide concrete experiences which children can understand and apply to more abstract situations. Handicapped children can learn most from multisensory learning experiences.

The final concern is to enhance communication, of which vocabulary development is an important aspect. Vocabulary developed through speech and signing can include movement. To help the student lacking speech development, the teacher can communicate visual experiences and encourage student expression through all appropriate means. Each class should expand vocabulary through pictures, discussions, questions and answers, texture cards, or creating music or sound scores, stories or poetry.

Words and ideas should be encouraged, attempts at communication, praised. The teacher's facial expression, dynamic use of voice, and complete involvement provides the catalyst for communication.

Effective teaching of handicapped children requires dedication, patience, love, and energy. It requires new teaching methods and materials to realize objectives for the class as a whole and for individuals. The teacher must be a flexible learner as well.

The teacher of creative movement is rewarded by students' change of expression, of interest, and abilities — such as the moment when an autistic child who previously refused all physical touch runs to give you a hug and dances out the room.

Creative movement works magic to which handicapped children should have access both as audience and participants.

References

Bender, Michael and Peter I. Valletutti, *Teaching the Moderately and Severely Handicapped*, Vol. I. Baltimore, MD: University Press. 1976,

Canner, Norma. *A Time to Dance*. Boston: Plays, Inc., 1975.

Cratty, Brayan, *Perceptual-Motor Behavior and Educational Processes*. Springfield, Illinois: Charles C. Thomas, 1969.

Doman, Glenn, *What to Do About Your Brain Injured Child*. New York: Doubleday & Company, Inc., 1974.

Grahan, Richard M., ed., *Music for the Exceptional Child*. Reston, Virginia: Music Educators National Conference. 1975.

L.S. Tsvetkova and T.M. Kuznetsova, "The Role of Visual Image and Perception in Speech Development of Children with Speech Pathology," *Journal of Special Education*, Vol. II, No. 3, New York: Greene and Stratton, 1977.

4 A Conceptual Framework for Teaching Dance to the Handicapped

Anne Riordan

Introduction

I have been working with persons with handicapping conditions for the last seven years and in that time there has been a natural evolution of my work and my ideas. I began with a small group of mentally retarded adults, and over the years as their skills progressed, this group formed the nucleus for Sunrise: a Special Dance Company, a company which has performed in over 20 cities in four states. With the addition of Sunrise Wheels, my group of wheelchair-bound adults, the group has expanded to include cerebral palsied individuals of normal intelligence and orthopedically handicapped.[1] Not all of my dancers perform with Sunrise or Sunrise Wheels for the group continues to grow in number, and it takes time to build the required performance skills.

Over the years, day to day my successes and failures have helped me develop some ideas which seem to work for me. The ideas developed naturally and intuitively, without intensive analysis. Only now, as I look back on the process to document it for this chapter, am I forced to bring an organized conceptual structure to it.

Writing is not easy for me, and I struggled for a long time to find an organizational framework on which to build my ideas about teaching dance to the handicapped. It was as if I were searching for a central theme for this "composition," just as I search for central themes for my dances for Sunrise and Sunrise Wheels. One evening, sitting down to indulge in a delectable French pastry, I thought, "Each of the layers of this pastry is good by itself, but combined, they are *exquisite*." The pastry, like my work with the handicapped, consists of many layers, each essential to the whole. I realized that I had used "layers" when speaking to groups about my work; using the "layer concept" to build this chapter seemed appropriate. After some thought and discussion with friends who know my work, I identified eight process layers in teaching dance to handicapped persons:

Physical Social
Emotional Spiritual
Psychological Creative
Intellectual Performance

These layers are synthesized with the content of each lesson through the teacher's skills and abilities. I shall discuss each area, beginning with the process layers, going on to the content base of the classes and the characteristics of the teacher, and finally presenting selected lessons which attempt to integrate theory and practice.

The Layers

Admittedly I do not consciously say "today I will deal with the intellectual or the physical layer." Each session is a natural combining of all of the layers with attention given to a specific layer as the need arises. In preliminary I identify the content, or the actual movement experiences, for that session. Being aware of and guiding the growth process on each of the layers happens in the session itself and it is a spontaneous response to the immediate situation. Layers overlap and intertwine in practice; only in theory can we separate them.

The Physical Layer

The physical layer attends the obvious need for strength, flexibility, stamina and endurance. Additionally it includes one need to develop an accurate body image and the kinesthetic awareness of the body's position and motion in space. In beginning sessions, this involves identifying body parts and spatial reference points such as front, back, side, high and low. As students absorb this information, they progress to more sophisticated body image and kinesthetic experiences.

---

[1] A film has been made documenting the work of this group. The title of the film is "A Very Special Dance" and it was produced by Judith Dwan Hallet and Karl Idsvoog of KUTV in Salt Lake City, Utah. The film has received numerous awards.

I must be aware of each individual physical limitation to encourage growth. But more than increasing strength or flexibility, growth includes increasing the participants' range of quality. Many of my students with limited movement repertoires consistently use familiar or "safe" movement patterns unless they are encouraged or challenged. When we talk about physical daring in the sessions, we deal with the strength and stamina necessary for performance, but just as often with the physical daring necessary to try new qualities of movement. *Courage*, whether to take the physical risk of maintaining a precarious balance with another person or the emotional/psychological risk of moving with entirely new patterns, is necessary to approach the unfamiliar.

The Emotional Layer

Many emotional factors allow a student to approach a session with daring and courage. It is essential to develop an effective *support system* in each group, whether from the teacher or from fellow group members. The members of Sunrise have been together a long time and at each performance I am amazed and delighted by the complexity and the subtlety of their support system. Aware of each other, they help each other get over the rough spots that inevitably arise in some performances. The support might be a touch, a look, or a smile, but the awareness and caring are always there if needed. Not only do they support each other, but they support me. No emotional relationship is a one-way process; my students support me as much as I support them.

One day, when I was feeling totally exhausted, one of the men rolled over to me in his wheelchair and said, "You look really tired, Annie. Why don't you sit down on my lap?" After he had convinced me that I wasn't too heavy and I had sat down gratefully, he said, "You really have to be more careful not to get so tired." One-way support? Never!

I value a support system. We talk about how important it is to know when someone else needs help, and we demonstrate and practice different ways of giving support. Equally important is knowing how to ask for support for ourselves. As strongly as I believe in giving and receiving support, there are times when it can get a little "mucky." There is a fine line between support and dependance. There are times when students need to be encouraged to pick themselves up and get on with the business at hand.

But the support system allows each individual to feel a sense of belonging. Belonging is another critical part of the emotional layer. Every person needs to belong and one important factor of that belonging is tolerance: tolerance of one's own limitations and those of others. Being accepted and valued in a group is important to every human being. Recently in one of the Sunrise rehearsals, the students were warming up, and I became involved with one student while the group started activity. Being occupied, I was unaware that one woman was not joining the group, but looked up to see another woman extend a hand and say, "Come on Mary, we *need* you in this dance." The gesture and the verbal invitation were familiar to me, for I have often used them in my own attempts to involve students in activity. Nevertheless, the effect of the invitation was touching and special. Mary got up with a shy smile and joined the group.

Acceptance, though vital, should not be confused with indulgence. When acceptance extends to inappropriate behaviors, such as tantrums, it becomes indulgence. Many of my students carry their emotions very close to the surface, and emotional outbursts are not uncommon. When this happens the teacher's role is to help the student regain *self control* and to deal with those strong emotions in socially acceptable ways. Time invested to help a participant regain self control is never wasted. The reader might think that when so much time is taken for one member of the group, the other members would become impatient. I'm not quite sure why, but members of my group are extraordinarily patient in these situations. Maybe there is an implied caring for each when I take time with one, or maybe they understand the feeling of being out of control and want to help too.

Each of these emotional factors, (giving and receiving support, belonging, tolerance, acceptance, and self-control) contribute to the success of the individual and the group. I cannot emphasize enough the value of success. Each time I see Sunrise or Wheels perform, the value of successful experiences radiates in the smiles and proud bows of the performers. Our audiences, also aware of the performers' pride, have communicated their delight in the joy and pride of the performers. While the emotional layer is critical, like the other layers in our pastry, it cannot stand alone.

The Psychological Layer

Involvement, responsibility for self, self-awareness and openness to new experiences are the elements of the psychological layer. These four psychological factors, dependent upon the physical and emotional factors discussed earlier, relate equally to the intellectual and social layers which follow. Probably every reader could define these four terms easily, yet the ability to define involvement or openness does not guarantee its achievement. The teacher must use all resources to set the psychological tone of each session; these qualities cannot be expected if they are not given. To a group I say, "Excite me! Thrill me! Dance means so much to me; show me what it means to you." I might demonstrate the difference between an involved performance and a detached performance and ask them to describe the difference. The teacher must *model* these psychological elements while accepting personal frailties. Yet the teacher need not be "Superman" or "Wonderwoman;" a "perfect model" — reassuringly — would be too much to handle. Modeling is nevertheless an effective way to set the tone of the sessions. Although it can be exhausting, the rewards are endless.

The Intellectual Layer

As a student participates in any new activity, regardless of content, vocabulary development ensues. Vocabulary development is a part of the intellectual layer of dance for the handicapped, but it is not the only nor even the most important part. Dance provides a unique opportunity for people to learn to "think on their feet." Remembering a sequence of movements while moving is a high level intellectual skill. In remembering and repeating a dance sequence, both long-term and short-term memory are employed. Dance experiences also develop concentration. The "short attention span" said to be characteristic of the handicapped may be true when activities are imposed on participants without attention to their interests. When the needs and interests are considered in the planning, the attention span becomes much longer. Concentration and attention span do not develop without time and patience. Whoever said, "The journey of a thousand miles begins with a single step," must have had taught handicapped persons.

Choice making is another intellectual aspect of dance for the handicapped. Making a decision based on a judgment is another high level intellectual skill. Improvising and/or choreographing provides many opportunities for choosing. Because I feel this is a very important skill, an outline of a "choice-making lesson" constitutes the last section of this chapter.

Vocabulary development, long and short-term memory, concentration, attention span, and choice making are only a few of the intellectual skills which can be developed through dance. Because I have found these factors central to my work, I identify them, but do not wish to exclude others.

The Social Layer

The handicapped frequently inhabit an egocentric world cut off from social interaction. It is, therefore, necessary for the teacher to identify acceptable and nonacceptable behaviors. Three guidelines are courtesy, cooperation, and responsibility (both for self and others). In addition to the obvious implications, I try to develop an awareness of others and an ability to identify with others. Dance offers a unique opportunity for experiences in cooperation (deciding together how to do a dance), responsibility (doing a dance which involves physically supporting another person's weight), and courtesy (watching patiently while others perform). Moving together in a shared experience can build a powerful foundation for understanding, mutual respect, and friendship.

The Spiritual Layer

I believe that dance has a special power to integrate the mind, body, and spirit. In aesthetic experiences the person can become whole, and thus can transcend self. I have heard that the handicapped don't need aesthetic experiences because they don't understand them, yet sometimes I think they understand better than the nonhandicapped. After Sunrise performances for modern dance majors at the University of Utah, I have been told that the dancers somehow touched the essence of dance. A graduate student once approached me after a Sunrise performance with tears in her eyes and said, "Thank you . . . thank you! I had forgotten . . . forgotten what dance could be!" If we cut handicapped persons off from aesthetic experiences, we chain them to their handicaps by not allowing them to go beyond themselves.

The Creative Layer

The creative process about which much has been written and little understood, is incredibly complicated. Creating in dance includes movement invention, combining movements, and forming dances. One does not begin the creative process with its most complicated part. I begin the creative process by encouraging awareness and expansion of one's own movement repertoire. These stages take time; only much later do we actually make dances. I do try to simplify the choreographic, however, and some of these procedures are included in the last section of this chapter.

The Performance Layer

Performance is an important part of the dance experience, and each of my sessions includes some performing—not with the lights, costumes, and props of a "fully produced" performance — but rather within time and space for an audience of one or more to sit and watch. Along with the performer's growth these experiences allow others to practice appropriate audience behaviors. At first, I set simple audience expectations such as quiet attention (or at least watching). I would perform for them when everyone complied. After my performances, I told them how good it felt to have everyone's attention. There were times, of course, when I had to stop, mid-performance, and reclarify expectations. Now reminders are rarely necessary.

The performance itself involves attention, concentration, focus, and self-discipline. The performers attend to directions and accompaniment, concentrate their energies to give their best performance, and focus on the task at hand to keep from being distracted by something as simple as an itching nose. Characteristic problems are not unlike those in any performance, except they are magnified somewhat. Waiting for the accompaniment to start without being distracted, making transitions without losing concentration, and holding the final position of a dance to indicate the ending are all critical in performances by handicapped and non-handicapped performers alike. Expectations must be identified and discussed if a good performance is to result.

Each layer discussed here carries equal importance in my sessions, although one may take priority or become the focus temporarily. But in the long run a balance of all of the layers is critical.

The Content

The content of dance classes, when based on the element of motion, provides endless combinations to serve as the core of each class. A general outline of activities, below, serves as the base for dance experiences.

I. Elements of Movement
    Time:
        consumed
        speed—fast, medium, slow
        body parts at different speeds
        altered speed
        stillness
    Energy:
        expended
        various amounts
        muscular tension or release of tension
        hard, soft, strong, weak, light, heavy
    Space and Shape:
        used self space (total body occupies)

        outside self space (place to move)
        direction, range, level
        forward, backward, sideward
        near, far, long, short
        high, medium, low
    Transition:
        point to point
        one movement to another
        free or bound
        one person to another
        beginning to end
II. Basic Movements
    Locomotor Skills
        crawl
        walk
        run
        jump
        hop
        leap
        slide
        gallop
        dodge
        roll
        skip
    Non-Locomotor Skills
        stand
        sit
        twist
        swing
        rotate
        stretch
        stop (freeze)
        bend
        turn
        pivot
        kick
III. Movement Problems—sensitizing with movements and movement elements
    Props — plastics, parachutes, wooden poles, balls
    Obstacle course—from the real to an obstacle course abstraction
    Music
    Partnering — men and women, trios, duets, and large groups
    Relaxation
IV. Choreography and Performance
    problem solving
    decision making
    choices

This outline, by no means complete, represents elements which may be included in a program. It is included to serve as a catalyst for ideas for other dance experiences.

The Conceptual Approach
to Movement Experiences in Dance

In teaching dance to the handicapped I have found that abstract movement experiences carry fewer stereotypes than literal experiences such as "be a tree," or "be a flower." Because literal movement experiences and their stereotypes seem to stifle inventiveness, I have focused my attention on non-literal, objective, or abstract movement problems. The elements of movement and the potential movements of the human body are the source of many student problems. For example, I might begin by asking students to shake their hands. Then the problem might extend to parts of the body, to shake the hands at different levels, to choose a place in space and freeze whenever the shaking part of the body got to that place, or to shake the hands where they cannot be seen, and so on. I think many beginning teachers have the opposite notion when they begin to plan lessons; thinking that imagery would be more stimulating, they are surprised that students are so responsive to the more abstract ideas. It has been my experience that the literal problems are not as effective as the conceptual or abstract ones.

The Role of the Teacher

I have skirted discussing the role of the teacher in this chapter. In discussing layers, I implied a role for the teacher, but this important issue warrants more attention. I have found some general characteristics and attitudes effective both in my own work and in training university students to work with my handicapped students. Desirable personality characteristics for working with handicapped persons include high energy level, enthusiasm, keen observation, the ability to involve self and others, willingness to take risks, openness to all situations, a positive attitude, honesty, expressiveness, and last, but definitely not least, a love of dance and an unquenchable desire to share that love with others. Some additional attitudes are critical.

First, the handicapped are not fragile; they do not have to be handled with kid gloves. While one must be aware of the natural limitations which the specific handicap imposes and set realistic expectations, that does not mean that the teacher should be overly protective. Over protection is neither needed nor wanted. Too often handicapped persons are babied and coddled like hot house plants. A realistic challenge, given with respect and understanding, comes as a welcome relief.

Second, the process is more valuable than the product. The focus and the dance experience is on involvement in movement for its own sake.

Perhaps my emphasis on performance seems to contradict my process focus. Yet the process of being involved in a performance is the goal which permeates my work. If a relatively polished performance (product) results, that's wonderful, but the primary focus is on the process. For this reason, Sunrise and Wheels performances intentionally include some preparation process, and are performed in the round rather than on a proscenium stage.

A final critical attitude is patience. Things take time. My university students who form their own groups are frequently frustrated by the tedious and time consuming work necessary in the beginning stages (and in the later stages, for that matter). Somehow they expect students new to dance to be able to do the things Sunrise does. I remind them that seven years work have built my students to where they are now. The teacher must be willing to approach each skill one step at a time and be satisfied by very small steps toward the goal.

Movement Experiences

In this last section certain movement experiences effective with my groups illustrate the braiding effect of the different layers with content. A few movement sessions are outlined:

1) A warm-up
2) Building to a choice-making lesson
3) Another choice-making lesson
4) A "responsibility for others" lesson
5) Guides to choreography

These lessons are taken from different skill levels. The warm-up can be used at almost any level and, in fact, each session includes some warm-up. The choice-making and responsibility for others lessons are more advanced and developed several years after I started working with my group.

1. A Warm-up Lesson

- In a circle, use gross motor activities to "wake up" large muscles of the body and get the "blood flowing." Be sure to spread out to avoid bumping.

Bend	These exercises can also be
Stretch	used to get the participants
Twist	"in gear" for the session to come
Reach	—a psychological and emotional
Shake	warm-up to go with the physical.

With beginning groups this experience helps assess the ability to follow directions, willingness to participate, and physical capacity. The subsequent tempo and content of the class can be geared to these assessments.

- Still in the circle, have students lie on stomachs and "swim," using both arms and legs. Assess natural opposition and ability to move in unfamiliar position.

- Using the swimming motion, have the students find a way to move into the center of the circle and back.
- Have students "swim on their backs" to the center of the circle and back out from the center.
- Come to a standing position, emphasizing the change of levels. Move to the center of the circle and back using changes of level, speed (fast and slow) and direction (forward and backward), adding as many variables as are reasonable.
- Build a sequence of directions reviewing the entire list each time a new direction is added. Perform that sequence.
- Continue adding to movements in and out of the circle while touching another member of the group with different parts of the body (hands, shoulders, elbows, hips etc.).
- Have students time their performance so that they all get to the center of the circle at the same time.

This warm-up session actually includes the physical, psychological, intellectual, creative, social, and performance layers. All of these layers intertwine with the content of the class under the guise of simply warming up the body.

2. Building to a Choice-Making Lesson

- With the participants standing in a circle, explain that when names are called the participants are to cross the circle in a straight line. (Lead up: have each participant hold his or her arm straight out in front and identify the person he or she is pointing toward, then walk straight to that person. This is difficult because of the round shape of the circle and the straight line of the movement).
- Model the behaviors desired.
- Make sure everyone knows where he or she will go.
- Call names one at a time, in a sequence around the circle so anticipation and preparation is possible.
- After everyone has crossed, repeat crossing but with names called in random order. It may be necessary to walk in front or beside some group members who have difficulty with this task. Warn participants that this will be harder, they will have to pay attention.
- Call names in random order and call more than one name at a time. Always explain and demonstrate every new set of directions. Deal with the possible "traffic" problem by showing how to slow down or speed up to avoid accidents.
- Warn that this next step is the hardest of all. Then tell them that each person must decide when he or she will cross the circle. Demonstrate with staff what happens when everyone goes at once (the circle disappears) and give some clues to help participants decide when to cross. Give individual attention to those who need it.

3. Another Choice-Making Lesson

- With the participants in partners, explain that one person will be the sculptor and will move the other person's body to different positions until "you really like the shape you have made." Demonstrate moving a partner and act out the decision making process while verbalizing it: "Hmmm. . . I don't think I like this position of George's head as well as the other one. I think I'll move it back."
- Give each partner a chance to be shaper/decider. Instruct the staff to circulate and help identify alternatives when someone in the group is having trouble.

This experience can lead directly into the following session.

4. Responsibility for Others Lesson

- After the shaping lesson, keep the same partners and face each other sitting down on the floor.
- Move together, mirroring each others' movement. Warn that it is necessary first to agree who will be the leader and who will be the follower.
- Explore different ways to move through space together without touching.
- Explore moving together while touching some part of the body.
- Explore supporting the weight of the partner's arms, being completely responsible for that weight. Add other parts of the body only when students comprehend the responsibility for each other.
- Eventually shift weight back and forth from one person to the other using verbal cues.
- Shift the weight back and forth from one partner to the other with no verbal cues.

I smile at how briefly this experience can be described. In reality, working through individual problems with each step in this sequence of development took months. This "responsibility experience" developed into the "Partner Dance" currently in the Sunrise repertory.

5. Guides to Choreography

The process of choreographing a dance takes many rehearsals to set the movement sequence. I choose a piece of music—frequently in the popular mode—which blends with the central theme of the dance. I emphasize to my students that the music can help "color their dance," and I ask them to show me that they are listening to the music. I set the stage by giving them the overall form of the dance, some "rules of the game." To a couple about to do a dance I might say, "This is a dance of friendship. You will start sitting on the floor apart from each other, stand, move toward each other, move together mirroring each others' movements, and then you will slowly sit down together." After reviewing the directions step-by-step with each partner, I would put on the music and let them try it. Then, just as all dancers receive feedback, we would sit and talk about what did and what didn't work. I might take one performer's role while the other dancer watches to illustrate some things to both dancers. This process of choreography is relatively high on the skill level continuum. Many modifications must be made for beginning dancers.

Making dances this way grows naturally from having time for performance in each session. But I must emphasize that students, some with seven years experience, model behavior for new members of Sunrise. Initially we choreographed with a very slow, step-by-step progression.

Conclusion

Now that the reader knows all of the ingredients for our "French pastry" it is time to go to the kitchen to try it. No "sure-fire recipe" has been given, simply because *there is none*. Starting with the basic ingredients, each "cook" must devise a special combination that "works." I wish you good cooking.

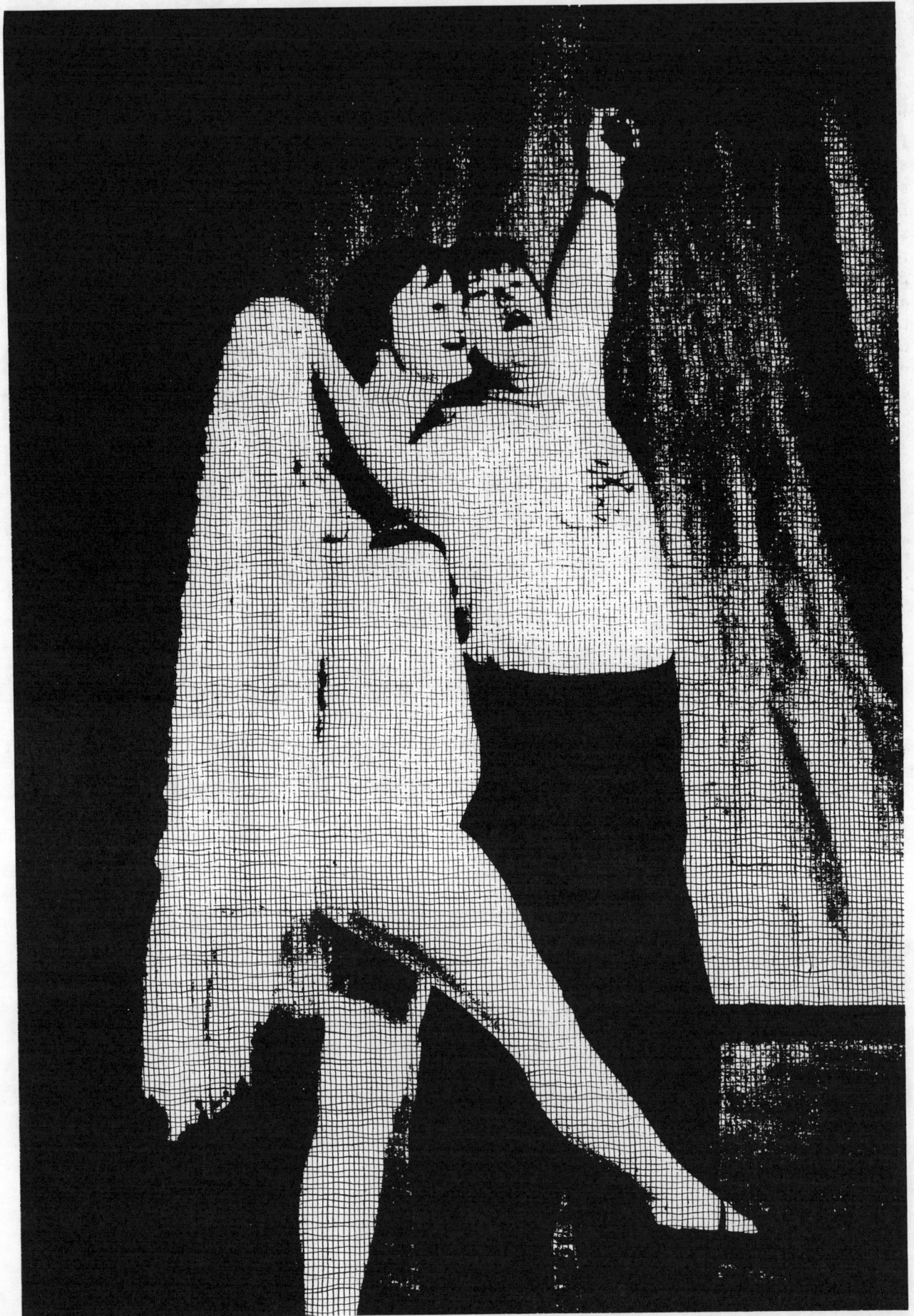

5 Anne's Magic

Sally Fitt and Anne Riordan

Introduction

Teaching handicapped persons involves much more than following a detailed lesson plan. The affective or emotional base one builds is just as important, if not more important, than the lesson content. Anne Riordan's preceding chapter presents some of the basic concepts she uses in teaching dance. Yet both Anne and I were concerned that her work might be reduced to simple lesson plans if we did not do an additional chapter on the "magic" or "art" of teaching. We realized that no art form can be fully analyzed and pidgeon-holed, but we wished to emphasize that the art of teaching is equally important as the conceptual base. We decided that it would be worthwhile to document, in some form, the "magic" essential to successful teaching of persons with handicapping conditions. We decided that I would observe Anne with different groups and try to identify non-verbal, affective behaviors and the patterns of verbal instructions to students. A number of observations formed impressions presented in the following chapter.

Identifying Components of the "Magic"

After observing Anne, I found myself with a volume of notes on her behavior in the sessions. Reviewing the notes, categories of behavior, "Anne's Magic," began to emerge: underlying assumptions, principles of teaching, verbal behavior, movement behavior, and affective behavior. Although the magic is more than the sum of these parts, an analysis of one successful teacher's behavior may provide insight into the teaching art. The categories overlap and no one could stand alone, yet they are analyzed separately for clarity.

Underlying Assumptions

Certain underlying philosophical assumptions are critical when working with persons with handicapping conditions. I found these assumptions guided almost every interaction Anne had with her students.

Anne is aware of the nature of each student's handicap and uses that knowledge in planning and adapting daily activities. She knows and accepts the limitations without limiting her students' growth, aware that a student growing beyond limitations needs support, encouragement, and guidance.

A delicate balance between acceptance and demand, both Anne and I feel, is the keystone of success. Demands on students must be realistic yet *nothing is impossible*. Who would have thought, when Anne started working with a small group of handicapped adults seven years ago, that her special dance company would perform all over Utah and in other states as well. *Nothing is impossible*. But without Anne's realistic and knowledgeable guidance in those daily sessions, the Sunrise Dance Company never would have developed.

Teachers must integrate realism (what is), pragmatism (what works), and idealism (what could be) in every interaction with students with handicapping conditions. Accepting, demanding, and reaching today beyond yesterday's dreams serve as the core of all work. The *balanced* combination of these three philosophical positions is essential to success. In other fields of teaching one can get away with a less balanced philosophical base. But with handicapped persons none of these assumptions can be ignored. Realism yields the acceptance of students, pragmatism guides growth, and idealism opens the possibility of achieving the impossible. The relative importance of these three assumptions shifts from day to day, but there must be a balance.

Application of the Principles of Teaching

Too often, teaching principles are left in the textbook when the teacher goes to class. Students may be required to learn in spite of the teacher rather than because of the teacher. Teachers of persons with handicaps cannot afford the luxury of ignoring teaching principles, for their students depend on them for motivation and guidance. In one group session, Anne used the following principles of teaching:

1) start where the students are;
2) clarify expectations;
3) ensure success;
4) positively reinforce appropriate behavior;
5) ignore inappropriate behavior;
6) consistently hold students to limits;
7) clarify when choices are appropriate and when they are not;
8) use visual, auditory, tactile, and kinesthetic senses;
9) modify expectations to meet individual needs.

The following section illustrates how Anne repeatedly used these principles.

Starting Where the Students Are

Arriving for the class, Anne checked with the staff to learn how her students were doing and was told one of the men was antagonistic, a "bad mood." It was interesting to watch Anne help him out of his mood, carefully designing successful experiences for him.

After everyone had changed into dance clothes, Anne entered to find some members of the group dancing to a record which one of the staff had put on the phonograph. Rather than stopping then starting the activity again, Anne joined the dance. She modified and developed what the dancers were doing so smoothly that students appeared unaware that the class had gone from improvisation with about half the group participating to directed activities with the whole group participating. Anne revised her lesson plan to effectively use the involvement she saw as she entered the studio.

Ensuring Success and Clarifying Expectations

Anne expertly insures the success of her students. She knows success is important, and uses every "trick" in the book to make sure students perform well. She repeatedly reviews expectations.

> "It would look terrific if your heads would all go up and down together."

Clarifying expectations is frequently accompanied by an "attention getter" or a gentle warning.

> "This is going to be hard so listen to me." "As soon as I get the record on I am going to come and check your circle. Make sure you aren't too close to each other. If you can touch the person next to you, you will have to adjust."

The warnings often take on the nature of a game.

> "Be careful now, I am going to try and trick you. You'll have to really listen for the signal."

It is clear that Anne will not accept less than the full attention and concentration of her students. But in making demands, she always restates her expectations, ensuring greater likelihood of success.

> "I am not putting the record on until all of you show me that you are ready. Your arms should be at your sides and you should be standing straight. No picking your nose or scratching your butt."

These are not idle threats. Since students know she really *does check,* they pay attention to her requests.

Positive Reinforcement of Appropriate Behavior

Once expectations are clearly outlined, Anne follows through and compliments her students. Sometimes she compliments the whole group, but just as often she compliments individual students who need special attention.

> "Oh my gosh, you've got it and it's fantastic." "That was terrific, Don, you really listened for the signal." "I was really worried where you all would get that, but it was beautiful. See, I got so excited, my watch fell off."

Ignoring Inappropriate Behavior

Anne's attention is a prize her students treasure. But sometimes the need for attention takes a negative course, and they test her to see if she will give them attention for misbehaving. Anne is incredibly able to ignore undesirable behaviors. At one point she was telling the students what to do next when one man picked her up, literally sweeping her off her feet. Without acknowledging the action in any way, Anne went right on giving instructions. Finding his play for attention had not been successful, the man put her back down. What followed this episode was as important as her ignoring the inappropriate behavior. As the man, behaving as was expected of him, moved off to join the group, Anne complimented him. Thus he gained the needed attention by positive rather than negative behavior.

Holding Students to Limits

Anne will not tolerate behavior that is less than students can manage. Not shy about demanding adherence to her standards, Anne becomes a five foot one inch master sergeant whose authority no student would dare challenge.

At one point in a session, as one of the most volatile men was about to leave the studio, Anne reminded him that he was to remain. Continuing to leave, Anne's behavior, movement, and tone of voice made it clear that she meant business.

Anne: "Over here, John!" (Accompanied by a straight, strong gesture).
John: "I'm just going out for a drink."

Anne: "Over here, right now!" (The gesture was repeated with greater intensity and a faster movement.)

John: "Well, okay."

Anne's demands for appropriate behavior are not always so strong and forthright. Many times, turning to a participant having difficulty managing in a group, she gently asks, "Are you going to be able to take control of yourself in this dance?" This is not an idle question. Anne waits for a response and appears willing to accept either a yes or no answer. If the answer is yes she makes sure that the participant understands the commitment by reidentifying the expectations. If the answer is no, which it seldom is, she would probably ask if the participant needed help.

Clarifying when Choices are Appropriate

Working in an art form which uses exploration as a tool sometimes encourages students to play with the dimensions of a movement. At other times, with a more specific goal, individual improvisation is not appropriate. Anne identifies which is expected.

"I want to see all new stuff here. No fair using things I've seen you do before."

"Let's see if we can really get it all together. Do you remember what came first?"

Working with Several Senses

Anne teaches as much by showing and doing as by telling. Visual and kinesthetic approaches reinforce the more traditional auditory method. She uses touch cues to help students get the feel of a movement. The multisensory approach gives students many different chances to understand directions.

Modification of Expectations

One day I watched Anne work with a group of fifteen children for the first time. Most were mentally retarded, but one boy had cerebral palsy and used a walker. After getting the children into a circle, she asked them to hold hands. The children next to the boy with cerebral palsy were instructed to hold the walker so the boy could hold the walker with his hands. She asked the children to shake their hands over their heads. Anne stood in front of the boy with cerebral palsy and encouraged him to hold the walker with one hand and shake the other over his head. Anne's sensitivity to the individual physical needs of her students extends to their emotional involvement. She is as likely to modify expectations for emotional as for physical reasons.

Verbal Behavior

Many examples in the teaching principles section illustrate effective patterns of verbal behavior. Effective in giving verbal instructions, Anne rapidly establishes key words and uses them to make understanding easier. Students come to understand that those words represent a whole cluster of behaviors.

Because Anne realizes that not all students have the same vocabulary, she repeats directions using different words. Verbal instructions are accompanied by showing what is expected so students may also key-in to non-verbal communication. Anne uses verbal directions more when she is working with a group. When she works one-to-one, non-verbal communication tends to predominate. Verbal directions to groups are clear and quite simple. She presents one component of the dance experience at a time, building each element on the preceding one. Adding to the sequence one step at a time, she is frequently able to encourage the participants to experience a relatively long dance sequence, with reminders about sequence throughout.

Anne's tone of voice indicates her expectations. Encouraging one student to try something never done before, her voice may be very soft, indicating her gentle support and understanding. For another student her encouragement might be quite firm. Anne's flexibility of tone encourages, stimulates, demands, shows acceptance, or reprimands. Her voice frequently communicates far more to the student than *what* she is saying.

Verbally expressing feelings is one of Anne's characteristics. She openly expresses delight or disappointment with her group. She seldom masks her own feelings, but rather is "up-front" to her students in words and actions. Her students love the sense of spontaneity this gives. Anne's verbal behavior, only one component of her success, is integrated with her knowledge of teaching, movement behavior, and affective behavior.

Movement Behavior

A wide range of movement behavior parallels Anne's use of her voice. Her flexible use of time, space, and force effectively meets situational demands, shifting dramatically as she works with different groups. Yet two common patterns are frequently repeated. Both the cluster of movement behaviors which encourage a student and those which hold a student to limits are central to Anne's success.

Movement Behavior to Encourage

When encouraging a student, Anne's characteristic movement behavior is slow, weak and curved. There are no surprises in her movement. The use of slow time gives the student time to see what she is doing. The low key weak force is gentle and unthreatening. The curved shape in space accomodates the student and implies acceptance. The use of physical contact — sometimes yielding, sometimes directing–but never controlling–is another nonverbal indicator of acceptance. Anne enters the student's personal space in a non-threatening manner. She frequently approaches the student from the side so that she can be seen, but she avoids eye contact as invasion of personal space combined with direct eye contact can be very threatening. The slow, weak approach gives the person a chance to move away, though this rarely happens. The sense of trust, established by the use of non-threatening movement enables Anne to build on and modify the movement she does with the student.

Holding a Student to Limits

Anne's movement behavior shifts quite dramatically when she is holding a student to previously established limits. In these instances her movements are usually slow and strong with a straight shape in space. The space and force components of movement changed but the slowness remains. Eye contact is direct, and her strong and straight posture and gestures make it clear that she means business. In these situations she frequently stands face to face with the student and maintains a firm physical contact. Often she places a hand on each side of the person's head and turns the head so that she can maintain direct eye contact. Although the touch appears firm, it somehow is also gentle, and one seldom sees anyone shying from it. Perhaps Anne is also vulnerable in these very close situations. She is putting herself on the line and students seem to know it and allow the close contact.

Anne's use of space changes more than the time component of her movement. She uses both direct, straight movements and indirect, curved movements, and varies the amount of space she uses. With an obviously shy and reticent participant, she uses smaller space and weaker force than with a

more eager participant. These nonverbal modifications to both situation and individual needs make participants more comfortable and help them grow without feeling threatened.

Affective Behavior

Anne sets a characteristically loving atmosphere in all of her sessions, yet there are many factors which contribute to the affective tone. Anne exhibits a constant sense of caring regardless of the situation. She respects the dignity of each student, encouraging the individual expression of each. Her sincerity and open caring does not allow students to be less than they can be. Her ability to rapidly establish trust in a group or one-to-one situation hinges especially on her willingness to take chances and expose her own vulnerability.

Anne's constant delight with movement contributes to the affective tone. She glows as she dances with her students and the glow is catching without being overwhelming. Anne takes care that her movements are within the capacity of her fellow dancers. She does not impose her own enthusiasm on students, but rather finds their own enthusiasm within them and magnifies it through her own. She openly "woos" her students and lets each participant know that he or she is very special to her. Adults, teachers and parents are frequently amazed by the level of participation Anne gets from students, even on first contact. After watching Anne in many different situations, I feel that she gets remarkable participation because of her open verbal and nonverbal expressions of trust, respect, joy, and love.

Conclusion

We have identified many components of Anne's behavior which may be central to her success with her students, yet none of them work alone. Anne's combination of elements is unique. Therefore, we do not identify these characteristics to give a prescription for success. These elements can be found in as many unique combinations and forms as there are skilled teachers of persons with handicapping conditions. Each teacher must find a personal style to incorporate the elements and find the magic and the art of teaching dance.

6 The Case for Dance for the Deaf

Aida Pisciotta

Dance education, long overlooked by many dance teachers, is ideally suited for and can be of even greater value to children who are deaf or profoundly hearing impaired. Creative dance taught by qualified dance teachers should be included in every school for the deaf in the country.

Briefly examining the education of the deaf child, we immediately encounter what is known as the "oral-manual controversy." The oral approach stresses speechreading and acquiring speech for communication, forbidding sign language other than natural gesture. The emphasis is on oral and written English. Proponents argue that the deaf should be able to understand and communicate within the hearing society. Opponents say that few deaf people become skilled enough at intelligible speech and speechreading to communicate freely with either the deaf or the hearing.

The manual approach, now usually taught as a part of the combined method, teaches American Sign Language (ASL) as the basis for communication. ASL is not directly translatable to English, though certain words which have no sign are spelled out with a manual alphabet called fingerspelling. Speech and speechreading skills are not stressed. Proponents argue that ASL is more appropriate than speech for the deaf, that the adult deaf community uses it, and that ASL users can learn to read as well as the orally trained. Opponents argue that ASL is not a complete language because it lacks both grammar and a written form, and further that the use of sign isolates the deaf within their own community.

The third approach, "total communication," or the combined method, uses speechreading, speech, ASL, and fingerspelling simultaneously and is supported by the National Association of the Deaf. The oral method and total communication are the two major approaches in use today.

The controversy centers around the concept of failure—failure of the method or of the child within the method. Manualists argue that the oral program prevents children from developing a natural and easy to use language, while incurring the frustra-

tion of trying to speak words few people understand and which cannot be monitored aurally. Oralists argue that users of sign are more deficient in reading because they lack practice in English for communication. They further argue that using ASL in conjunction with English, as in total communication, makes the deaf reluctant to attempt and practice speech because their peers more easily understand signing. Whatever the method, "from all available evidence, even a moderate criterion of success, such as a reading level of better than grade four, is only achieved by about 25 percent of all deaf children when they finally leave school after twelve or more years" (Furth 1973). According to these standards at least, most deaf children continually experience failure and the frustration caused by it throughout their school years.

To help overcome the insecurities failure causes, children need experiences, such as creative dance, in which success is intrinsic. Margaret Murrel (1959) speaks of a dance program at Arkansas School for the Deaf: "Visually hearing his audience's approval and emotionally feeling his successful participation in a group routine bring self-confidence to a deaf child and increase his desire to speak and act naturally among those in the hearing world."

Dance should be taught to deaf children for many of the same reasons as to hearing children. Ruth L. Murray (1975) writes "Probably the first reason children need to dance is that they have a hunger for movement which must be satisfied if their proper biological development is to be achieved." Familiarity with and control in body movement aids total development. "Control of one's own body can mean the beginning of self-control in general. Having controlled this most obvious part of his environment, control of temper and other emotions are, for most people, easier" (Breckenridge and Vincent 1965). All children benefit from dance as a form of creative expression because

dance provides a primary medium for expression involving the total self, not just a part, like the voice, or totally separated from the physical self, like painting or sculpture. Dance and the movement that produces it is

25

'me,' and as such, is the most intimate of expressive media. A child's identity, self-concept, and self-esteem are improved in relation to such use of the body's movement. (Murray, 1973).

That dance expression is particularly appropriate for the deaf becomes clearer when we examine the specific circumstances of deafness. The sense of hearing serves in a nondirectional, signaling manner and constantly informs the organism of changes in the environment (Myklebust 1960). In contrast to vision, hearing is ever present and cannot be turned off, even during sleep. *Only when one is fully cognizant of this uniqueness of hearing can one understand the extreme isolation which occurs from deafness*" (Myklebust: author's italics). In comparison with the normal child, studies of deaf children show they are deficient in total life experience.

Where verbal ability is a factor, the deaf, understandably, are found to be inferior to the hearing in tests of mental ability. In cases where language facility is not important, this is not always true; in fact, in some tests the deaf are found to be superior to the hearing. Blair (1957) used the Knox Cube Test to test memory for movement patterns. Myklebust describes this test as a measurement of an individual's ability to observe, organize, retain, and reproduce movement patterns. The vision and tactual-kinesthetic sensory associations, make it a visuo-motor-kinesthetic problem for deaf children (Myklebust). Blair found that deaf children scored significantly higher than their hearing counterparts. Myklebust suggests that the visual perceptual processes develop differently in the profoundly deaf because the deaf "are dependent on visual clues which are irrelevant when hearing is normal". Blair also found deaf children superior to the hearing on design memory test. While the hearing tried to remember the design by associating it with something in their experience, the deaf merely observed and reproduced.

These findings have tremendous implications for dance for the deaf. Dr. Peter Wisher, who has been working with deaf adults in creative dance at Galludet College says, "Dependence on the visual serves to emphasize the importance of movement, which is an important aspect of communication. . . . Consequently, the area of the dance might have relatively more importance in the lives of the deaf than on the hearing." Because movement is language for the deaf, whether of the lips speaking or the hands signing, it follows that they should have as much movement experience as possible. If deaf children have a special aptitude for recognizing and remembering shapes and movements, then dance, which involves those elements, should be

encouraged. I have found that for all but one of the six deaf children I have been teaching in Salt Lake City skills needed for dance come very naturally. They have remarkable memories for their own dance compositions. When I ask them to recall a sequence which they created weeks before and have not practiced since, they can do it quite well. When learning movement sequences they are attuned to minute details of movement, such as, whether the palm faced up or down, or whether the head nodded just before or after a shoulder shrug. Trained dancers sometimes fail to notice such particulars. If deafness enhances the visual and kinesthetic senses, most important in dance, then deaf children should have dance experiences in order to develop to their full potential as human beings.

I am not suggesting that we train deaf children to be professional dancers. Rather, we should enrich their sensorily deprived lives by maximum stimulation of the remaining senses through dance as an art form. Exposure to the arts helps children to become more well-rounded individuals. A. H. Maslow (1971) states "the goal of education . . . is ultimately the 'self-actualization' of a person, the becoming fully human, the development of the fullest height . . . that the particular individual can come to." He adds "It happens that music and rhythm and dancing are excellent ways of moving towards the discovery of identity." He speaks of this as "intrinsic education" which would "have art education, music education, and dancing education as its core. (I think dancing is the one I would choose first for children. . . .)"

Creative dance experiences provide opportunities for socialization lacking in deaf schools. Working in partners or groups to explore movement problems, children learn to respect each other's ideas and to come to a cooperative solution. A sensitive teacher could combine deaf with hearing children at times, giving them the opportunity to work closely with their hearing peers. This opens more mainstreaming possibilities to deaf children.

The most direct effect of deafness is restricted communication. Whether they speak or sign, the deaf must feel frustration and insecurity in trying to communicate, especially with the hearing. Yet deaf people are physically very expressive, since they often rely on gestures and facial expression to be understood. The frustration of verbal communication can be alleviated by providing nonverbal, physical expression through dance.

Each child in the creative dance class is guided to develop creative potential, participating in an activity in which deafness is no handicap. Two of the children in my class have more hearing than the others, yet succeed no more than their classmates. Probably the most creative boy in the class one who consistently creates interesting dance studies and dances with quality, is the youngest and the most profoundly deaf.

Besides being a satisfying outlet for expression, dance calls upon the very skills essential to effective speechreading and speech. The person who can speechread well can often read and speak well. Myklebust explains that the deaf child acquires speech and his inner language visually but monitors speech through his tactual-kinesthetic sense. "This need to . . . shift from one monitoring system to another in learning language . . . may be one of the most difficult problems in learning encountered by Man!" A person who learns and performs dance movement learns the movement through vision, then monitors performance of it through the kinesthetic sense. Practice in learning and performing dances, in addition to being satisfying to the individual, helps perfect skills needed to speechread and speak. For this reason deaf children need to learn movement as well as to create their own. Having children teach each other movements they have created has the additional benefit of giving the teaching child a feeling of importance and practice in leadership skills.

The value of rhythm as it pertains to speech in deaf education has long been recognized; many deaf schools have some type of rhythm program. Deaf people often speak in a rhythmical monotone, a characteristic which contributes to the unintelligibility of their speech. Rhythmic training helps improve this aspect of speech. Sandra Hagen, who taught creative dance at Callier Speech and Hearing Center in Dallas, used dance as a stimulus to aid deaf children with speaking problems. In *Dance in a Silent World* (1971) Hagen explains that when language and movement go together, children can learn the rhythm of a word by moving to it.

Deaf children can increase their verbal vocabulary through dance by "dancing the words." They can learn words such as "tension" and "relaxation" by physically experiencing them. The children rarely forget vocabulary they have learned through a pleasant dance experience.

Teaching dance to the deaf is similar to teaching the hearing. Students should understand the aesthetics and elements of dance so that they can express themselves creatively. Approaches to dance which rely heavily on vision are successful with the deaf. The dance teacher who cannot rely on music to carry the lesson may feel handicapped at first yet children can feel some vibrations through

the floor. In nearly every deaf class a few children can sense a beat in music, especially the deep bass in rock and roll. Other children soon learn to cue visually from the others, sensing the beat kinesthetically as they move.

I noticed that the children in my fifth grade deaf class, perhaps because of the lack of sound distraction, seemed able to concentrate better and longer than hearing children. They have a different sense of duration than I do; they can create a dance study five or more minutes without feeling it may be too long to do or to watch. Intensely physical, they are often hyperactive. They have a strong need for positive reinforcement, often asking "Who was better?" even though I explain that there is no "better" or "worse," only different. Most strikingly, the children did not have the conventional biases of hearing children. In my class of five boys and one girl, none of the boys was reluctant to dance, even at first. They had never heard that dancing is for girls, or that boys who dance are "sissies."

It seems clear that deaf children have a special need to dance. With the uphill struggle to learn language throughout their schooling, self-expressive relief within this nonverbal, physical art form provides is important. The sensory deprivation which results from profound deafness is compensated for by maximum stimulation of the remaining senses. Insecurities caused by the lack of normal language skills disappear in the dance classroom. Creative dance expression provides a much needed contribution to the total education of the deaf child.

References

Blair, F. "A Study of the Visual Memory of Deaf and Hearing Children." *American Annals of the Deaf*, 96, 502, 1951.

Breckenridge, M. E., and Vincent, E. L. *Child Development*. 5th ed. Philadelphia: Saunders, 1965.

Edwards, E. M. *Music Education for the Deaf*. South Waterford, Maine: The Meriam-Eddy Co., 1974.

Furth, H. G. *Deafness and Learning, A Psychosocial Approach*. Belmont, California: Wadsworth Publishing Co., Inc., 1973.

Giangreco, C. J., and Giangreco, M. R. *The Education of the Hearing Impaired*. Springfield, Illinois: Charles C. Thomas, 1970.

Hagen, Sandra. *Dance in a Silent World* (MFA thesis). Dallas: Southern Methodist University, 1971.

Maslow, A. H. *The Farther Reaches of Human Nature.* New York: Penguin Books, 1971.

Murray, R. L. A Statement of Belief. In G. Andrews Flemming, ed. *Children's Dance.* Washington D.C.: AAHPER Publications, 1973.

Murray, R. L. *Dance in Elementary Education* (3rd ed.). New York: Harper and Row Publishers, Inc., 1975.

Murrel, Margaret. "Dance for the Deaf Child." *Journal HPER,* 30, 7, 1959.

Myklebust, H. R. *The Psychology of Deafness.* New York: Grune and Stratton, 1960.

Whetnall, E., and Fry, D. B. *The Deaf Child.* Springfield, Illinois: Charles C. Thomas, 1964.

7 Creative Movement for the Young Hearing-Impaired Child

Rebecca I. Reber

First, young children are at the stage where they learn directly from personal experience and action. Their knowledge of themselves comes from personal experience and experiment in movement.

—Russell (1975)

Like other children, young hearing-impaired children develop awareness of self, time, space, and force in a creative movement class and begin to manifest creative behaviors. A controversy exists as to whether or not hearing-impaired children are as creative as children with normal hearing. Johnson and Khatena (1975) and Singer and Lenahan (1976) show that deaf children score significantly lower than their hearing peers when verbal tests are used to assess creativity. In a study by Rogers (1976) and three studies by Silver (1977), however, it was found that when nonverbal instruments assess creativity, deaf children do not lag behind their hearing peers. Rogers and Silver used the Torrance Tests of Creative Thinking with Pictures, Form P, and Figural Form A (Torrance 1966), respectively, as nonverbal assessments of creativity. In addition, Silver used panels of judges to assess drawings and paintings produced in experimental art classes.

In support of creative movement exploration for all children, Torrance (1965) found that the fluency, flexibility, and originality aspects of creative thinking greatly improved after participation in a creative movement class. Important to every child, creativity should be encouraged and given the opportunity to grow.

This paper is based upon a year's work with children of moderate to severe hearing impairment, ages four to seven, from the Denton Regional Day School Program for the Deaf, Denton, Texas. Children were transported twice weekly, to the Texas Woman's University gymnasium for 50 minute sessions of guided creative movement. Total communication, with reliance upon demonstration and manual prompting, was used in these sessions since both the staff and children exhibited varying levels of signing proficiency.

Needs of Young Hearing-impaired Children

Creative movement classes, like other instructional areas, should begin with an assessment of the children's needs and/or behaviors. Observation, the use of rating sheets, and interviews with classroom teachers showed the hearing-impaired children to have the following special needs which could be met by guided creative movement: (1) gross body coordination, (2) rhythm skills, (3) expressive body communication, (4) spatial awareness, (5) balance skills, (6) body awareness, and (7) group awareness and socialization skills. The methods discussed in the remainder of this paper were used to meet these needs.

A Framework for Teaching Movement

The Texas Woman's University (TWU) creative movement program for deaf children derives basic concepts from the work of Rudolf Laban, well known for his analysis of movement, and Joan Russell (1975) who has adapted Laban's concepts to young children. The following themes form the basis of the TWU creative movement program for deaf children:

Theme 1. Concern with awareness of the body (body aspect)

Theme 2. Concern with awareness of force and time (effort aspect)

Theme 3. Concern with awareness of space (space aspect)

Theme 4. Concern with awareness of the flow of body weight in time and space (effort aspect)

Theme 5. Concern with adaptation to partners (relationship aspect).

When structuring lessons for children, these Themes are age-related. Themes 1, 2, 3, and 5 are suggested for five to six year olds. The same Themes are expanded for six to seven year olds with the addition of Theme 4. Theme 1, body awareness, for five to six year olds, includes activities which involve the whole body in stepping and running, spinning and turning, galloping and skipping, locomotion on all fours, and leaping, hopping, and jumping. Body awareness also includes exploring possible actions of the hands and feet, such as beating on the floor, grasping and releasing objects, and kicking and shaking. Body awareness for six to seven year olds, includes experiences of spreading and shrinking, rising and sinking, and one introduction of other body parts, such as the knees and elbows.

Themes 2 and 4, dealing with the effort aspect, include activities for experiencing quick and slow speed variations, and weight in the strength of hands against each other or feet pushing into the floor, contrasted with activities such as light-footed stepping. Additional effort material for six to seven year olds includes experiencing gradual and rapid changes in speed and weight.

Space, Theme 3, explores near and far space in directions of above, in front, sideways, on the ground, and behind. Use of body parts to lead movements in space, use of straight, twisted or curved pathways, and use of high, medium and deep levels add challenge for the six to seven year olds.

Theme 5, relationship, involves the five to six year old child working as an individual with the whole group and in relationship to the teacher. The six to seven year old is generally ready to experience action/reaction with a partner, and work in groups of three, or in larger groups following a leader's actions.

Movement Songs

Wisher (1974), an authority in dance for the deaf, suggests that spoken language deficiencies related to deafness made dance training significant in the learning process. Deaf children can learn many new words through movements expressing poems, songs, and stories. Movement/dance songs provide a total group affinity and have been identified in the guidelines developed by the Task Force on Children's Dance (AAHPER, 1973) as being important to a comprehensive dance curriculum. For hearing-impaired children, action songs have been found to develop and improve body-image (Galloway and Bean 1974).

Fleming (1976) discusses the use of dance songs to facilitate movement, foster creativity, and provide varied rhythmic experiences. Singing and dancing about what, how, and why people move can be developed by individual or groups of children, as well as teachers and other adults working with children. The movement songs require exploring, identifying, inventing, and improving movement qualities. By singing and dancing out ideas, understandings are reinforced.

Fleming lists many purposes of movement songs. The following are just a few which can be applied to work with the hearing-impaired: getting movement started, increasing kinesthetic awareness, having fun together, involving all in participation, assuring accomplishment for all, sensing and responding, thinking and problem solving, quieting a group down after overstimulation or exhilaration, reinforcing concepts and learning, and initiating a creative experience. Fleming suggests that among traditional movement songs the best enable teachers to capture children's spontaneous experiences in creative rhythmic movement activities.

Props

In a dance setting for hearing-impaired children, props provide a mood, teach movement concepts, stimulate movement, encourage shy children, create security, and allow creative and imaginative play. Delaney (1979) discusses the use of soft materials, such as nylon fabrics of different hues for children to wrap up in, to move with, to feel, and to use in imaginative play. Soft stretchy tubular knit fabrics may be used for hammocks, for bouncing into, for being inside or while experimenting with shape making, and for dramatic play and fantasy action.

Dress-up clothes, scarves, and balloons help explore new movement qualities, expand movement repertoire, and encourage expressive body use. Balloons and scarves can be used to stimulate movement or to teach one light/heavy aspects of effort. Deaf children can also feel the vibrations of music being played by holding balloons. Dress-up clothes allow the children to cast off inhibitions and expand and exaggerate previously restricted movements.

Relaxation

To bring children to a quieter state at the close of the movement session, relaxation should be integral to the creative movement time. Delaney illustrates how (Sherrill, 1976) soft fabrics can facilitate relaxation. Fleming (1976) suggests using associations and feelings to help children relax the whole body.

Conclusion

Developing creative behaviors in children with hearing impairments can be facilitated with the same concepts and teaching techniques as with other children. In working with deaf children, however, the teacher's expressive body language to communicate, movement songs to enhance the children's language skills, and creative movement concepts to allow expression of inner emotions and encourage creative behaviors are especially important.

References

Children's Dance. Gladys A. Fleming, ed. Reston, Virginia: American Alliance for Health, Physical Education, and Recreation (AAHPERD), 1973.

Delaney, Wynelle. "Fabrics, Balls, and Pillows in Dance and Movement Discovery" in *Creative Arts for the Severely Handicapped.* Claudine Sherrill, ed. Springfield, Illinois: Charles C. Thomas, 1979.

Delaney, Wynelle. "Dance Therapy and Adapted Dance," in *Adapted Physical Education and Recreation.* Sherrill, Claudine. Dubuque, Iowa: Wm. C. Brown Co., 1976.

Fleming, Gladys A. *Creative Rhythmic Movement.* Englewood Cliffs, New Jersey: Prentice-Hall, 1976.

Galloway, H. F. and Bean, M. F. "The Effects of Action Songs on the Development of Body-Image and Body-Part Identification in Hearing-Impaired Preschool Children." *Journal of Music Therapy,* 11, 1974, pp. 125-134.

Johnson, Roger and Khatena, Joe. "Comparative Study of Verbal Originality in Deaf and Hearing Children." *Perceptual and Motor Skills,* 40, 1975, pp. 631-635.

Laban, Rudolf. *Mastery of Movement.* L. Ullman, ed. London: Macdonald and Evans, 1960.

————— . *Modern Educational Dance.* Rev. by L. Ullman. London: Macdonald and Evans, 1963.

Rogers, Terry, "The Role of Education in the Development of Creative Abilities of Deaf and Hearing Children, Ages Five and Eleven." *Texas Journal of Audiology and Speech Pathology,* 1976, pp. 8-10. Reviewed in Ellen Lubin. "Motor Creativity of Preschool Deaf Children." Doctoral dissertation, Texas Women's University, 1978.

Russell, Joan. *Creative Dance in the Primary School.* London: Macdonald and Evans, 1975a.

————— . *Creative Movement and Dance for Children.* Boston: Plays, 1975.

Silver, Rawley A. "The Question of Imagination, Originality, and Abstract Thinking by Deaf Children." *American Annals of the Deaf,* 1977, 122, pp. 349-354.

Singer, D. C. and Lenahan, M. L. "Imagination Content in Dreams of Deaf Children." *American Annals of the Deaf,* 1976, 121, pp. 44-48.

Torrance, Paul E. "Seven Guides to Creativity." *Journal of Health, Physical Education and Recreation.* 1965, 36, pp. 26-27.

————— . *Torrance Tests of Creative Thinking.* Princeton: Personnel Press, 1966.

Wisher, Pete. "Therapeutic Values of Dance Education for the Deaf." *Dance Therapy.* American Alliance for Health, Physical Education, and Recreation. C. R. Mason, ed. Reston, Virginia: AAHPERD 1974.

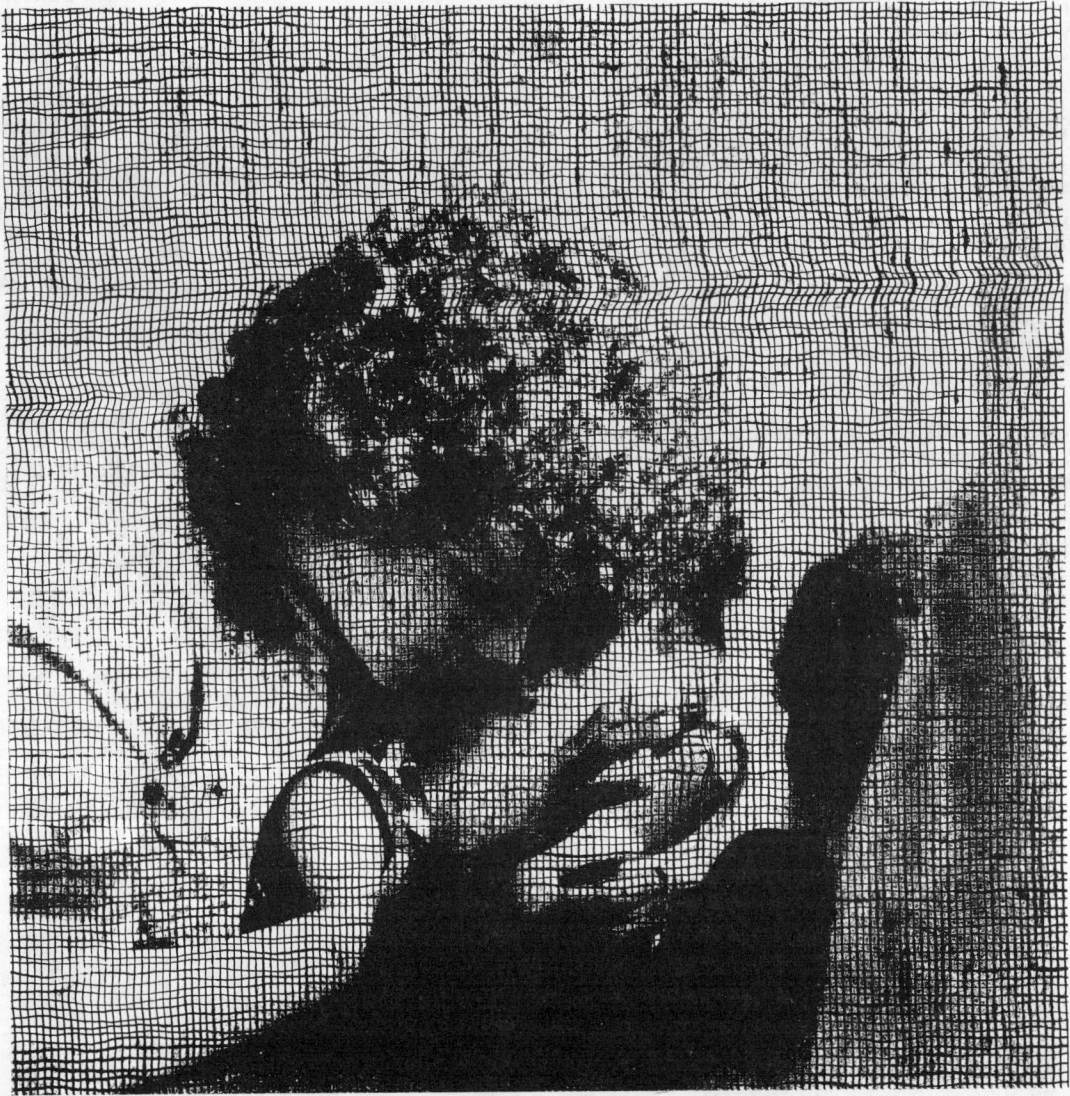

8 Dance/Movement Communication for Young Deaf Adolescents

Carol Kay Harsell

. . .Throughout the span of human existence, dance has been a part of the life of every tribe, society, and culture. It is one way humans have invented to express their essence. In primitive societies, people danced to eliminate evil spirits, to bring in crops, and to ask for rain. In modern societies, people still dance to express their joy and exuberance and banish their cares.

from ''Dance as Education''

Because it is rooted in natural functions, dance movement provides way for the deaf child to communicate feelings and to integrate inner and outer worlds. Deafness may retard language acquisition, thereby limiting the child's ability to express thoughts and feelings. Authorities agree that the primary handicap of deafness is the limitation imposed on communication (Wisher 1974, Sherrill 1976; Myklebust 1964).

Dance/creative rhythmic movement is recognized as one of the best ways to help children learn to communicate (Fleming 1976; Lockhart 1977. Murray 1963). Dr. Peter Wisher of Gallaudet College in Washington, D.C. has shown that deaf university students can communicate ideas and thoughts to hearing audiences through the medium of modern dance. He has described methods for teaching dance to young adults in several articles. Little, however, has been written on methods of teaching dance to younger deaf adolescents.

The ideas and methods presented in this article are based on work done with 32 young adolescents at the Denton Regional Day School for the Deaf, Denton, Texas. While the hearing loss varies in these youngsters, all had problems great enough to warrant educational placement separate from their hearing peers: five wore hearing aids, and one ado-

Figure 1. Harsell Core/Flexibility Design for Teaching Dance to Deaf Adolescents

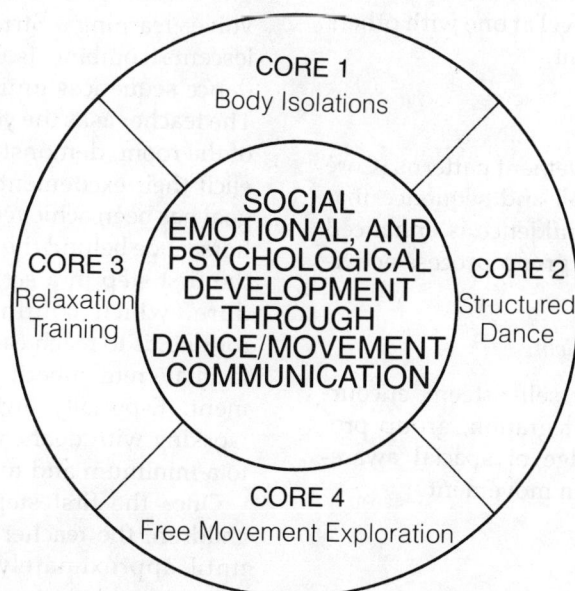

CORE 1
Body Isolations

CORE 3
Relaxation Training

SOCIAL EMOTIONAL, AND PSYCHOLOGICAL DEVELOPMENT THROUGH DANCE/MOVEMENT COMMUNICATION

CORE 2
Structured Dance

CORE 4
Free Movement Exploration

lescent had partial hearing. Five percent of the adolescents were only able to feed vibrations in their body with maximum music volume. The adolescents' speech abilities were limited. The focus of their communicative ability was signing, eight of the group had limited speech ability.

The Harsell Core/Flexibility Design

The method of teaching dance to these deaf adolescents has been designated as the Harsell Core/Flexibility Design: a Supplemental Educational Plan. This method, first developed and used with normal children and adolescents, was also found effective after 12 weeks of experimentation, with deaf adolescents.

The Harsell Core/Flexibility Design can be visualized as a circle within a circle (see Figure 1). The inner circle is the core of the program; the outer circles reflect the flexibility and creativity one shares with individual children in teaching communication or ideas and feelings through dance/creative movement. The components of the core are described below.

Central Core: Social, Emotional, and Psychological Development Through Dance/Movement Communication

Core 1 Body Isolations:

Slowly, each part of the body is individually explored as to the movement possibilities, shapes, rhythms, and directions which help integrate the inner and outer world of the self. The goal is to develop a natural positive sense for movement and to help the child interact and feel at one with others and nature through movement.

Core 2 Structured Dance:

This phase reinforces the movement patterns (Core 1) through his ability to recall and sequence that which has been learned. Confidence is enhanced while engaging in social and group process activities.

Core 3 Free Movement Exploration:

This phase builds confidence, self- esteem, encourages sensory stimulation, integration, group process, socialization, knowledge of spacial awareness, creativity, and efforts in movement.

Core 4 Relaxation Training:

This phase develops an awareness of inner rhythm, the ability to slow down the circulatory system, produce a healthy mental attitude through elimination of stress and lengthening the attention span to facilitate learning.

The four core areas the dance educator working with deaf adolescents. The Harsell Core/Flexibility Design is *flexible* in that the interchangeable cores are used at different times and speeds depending upon the group.

Body Isolations

A typical dance session with deaf adolescents begins (Core 1) by teaching them to feel comfortable with a new form of expression: their body in motion. The children remove shoes and socks to maximize vibratory input from the floor, and form a circle to ensure teacher visibility and to enhance a feeling of unity. Slowly the adolescents are led through a series of movements, starting with the head and working down the body to the toes. The adolescent experiences standing, sitting, lying down, rolling, and other movement patterns in various rhythms established by the teacher with the aid of a drum. After this brief introduction each student is given the opportunity to serve as leader, while the others follow. The flexible teaching method permits each student to participate in unique manner while adhering to the original Core 1-Body Isolations. The teacher may invent other ways to explore body isolations as the students become familiar with what is expected in this activity.

Structured Dance

The second part of the dance session (Core 2) involves learning a Structured Dance. Here the adolescents combine isolated body movements into dance sequences until a finished product evolves. The teacher asks the young people to sit on one side of the room, demonstrating enough of the dance to elicit their excitement and enthusiasm. When this goal has been achieved, the students form lines or a horseshoe behind the teacher as the teacher teaches the first step in a series. The object of this procedure, which continues throughout the dance routine, is to teach each step in its simplest form to facilitate remembering and reproducing the movement. Especially important considerations when working with deaf children are to keep frustration to a minimum and to ensure greatest success.

Once the first step has been mastered by the children, the teacher introduces subsequent parts until approximately one quarter of the dance routine has been taught. At this point it is good to divide the children into fours and twos for small group practice and performance. When the groups demonstrate command of this part of the routine, the teacher instructs the next quarter of the dance and proceeds until the dance is completed. The time spent on Structured Dance depends on the class and the objectives of the teacher, but for positive results this portion of the class generally lasts no more than 20-25 minutes of an hour session.

During the Structured Dance session the deaf child cannot hear the dance instructor counting the beat nor giving movement instructions. This problem is intensified when the teacher does not face the group as often happens in executing dance steps which involve changes of direction. As a consequence, it is necessary to devise a method of communication which does not depend upon sound and speech reading. This can be accomplished by shining a flashlight on the wall the children face. The light shows direction of movement, lessens confusion, and helps the children to count the beats for themselves.

The dance music rhythm is communicated by hand signals to children who cannot hear, such as a continuous flexion and extension of the wrist in time to the music. Once cued visually, most deaf children are able to capture and maintain the beat kinesthetically. The teacher may then employ the technique of fading. The hand signals, given first from the front, then from the side of the room are gradually lessened until total fading occurs. It may be necessary to repeatedly remind deaf children to watch for cues. As they may manifest their desire for independence by insisting they do not need help, remind them to watch for the *rhythm*, not because they do not know the dance.

Free Movement Exploration

Free Movement Exploration (Core 3) emphasizes developing the pupil's creativity. It is important for everyone, including deaf adolescents, to express and vent emotions in group situations and alone in a positive, constructive manner. Creativity is not a gift given to a select few. Creative behaviors are learned through teaching methods which encourage a person to explore inner and outer worlds. Stimulating the existing visual, kinesthetic and tactile senses teaches the deaf adolescent to satisfy, express, and expand communication of thoughts and feelings through dance movements.

Slides, film, and pictures are excellent stimuli for movement communication. Flashing a scene on the wall can encourage a particular mood about which the pupil selects one movement to portray an evoked feeling. A second, third, and fourth movement are added and blended into a final composi-

tion, either alone or within a group. The deaf adolescent who becomes more familiar with experiencing and interacting, with different sights and feelings, communicates better through movement and feels more secure.

During the Free Movement Exploration time, props and objects stimulate visual, kinesthetic, and tactile senses, while teaching the interrelationships of space, force, and time.

Relaxation Training

At the end of every dance session Relaxation Training (Core 4) takes place in a large circle in the middle of the room. Adolescents are led in swaying motions beginning with the head and trunk, followed by the arms. Slowly all descend to the floor and lie prone with arms and feet outstretched for approximately five to ten minutes.

Although this part of the session may sound insignificant, deaf pupils, often extremely restless, may suffer from a great deal of stress. The adolescent who cannot learn to control the rhythms of this own body, may be increasingly hampered.

General Suggestions for Teaching Deaf Adolescents

Other suggestions which may prove helpful to the dance educator in working with deaf adolescents follow. To attract pupils' attention, speak to the total group or begin a new series of events, flick the lights off and on. When switching from core to core, changing line formations helps the adolescent understand that the next phase is to take place and enhances continuity and security in the dance lesson.

With the pupils' backs to the light, the teacher should speak normally and directly at eye level while concurrently using sign language. If the teacher does not command sign language, a simple sign language course is helpful. Teaching dance to a deaf adolescent holds the same frustrations and promise as to any other child. Except for the few differences mentioned, the deaf adolescent is generally cooperative and athletic, has an excellent memory, and is eager to learn. Communicating with the deaf child is a cooperative effort; the major barrier is lack of effort on either side.

Deaf pupils, as all persons need to be accepted, respected, and given the tools for growth. The ego needs protection during a child's formative years. It is the role of every educator to ensure every child the most fun with the least amount of damage to facilitate optimal emotional, social, and psychological development.

References

Avery, C. B. "The Education of Children with Communication Disorders" in Education of Exceptional Children and Youth, Cruickshank, Wm. M. and Johnson, C. O., eds. Englewood Cliffs, New Jersey: Prentice-Hall, Inc., 1975.

Dance As Education. Reston, VA: National Dance Association. AAPHER, 1977.

Gilliom, B. B. *Basic Movement Education for Children*. Reading, Massachusetts: Addison-Wesley Publishing Co., 1970.

Lockhart, A. and Pease, E. *Modern Dance Building and Teaching Lessons*. 5th ed. Dubuque, Iowa: Wm. C. Brown, 1977.

Murray, R. L. *Dance in Elementary Education*. New York: Harper and Row, 1973.

Myklebust, H. R. *The Psychology of Deafness, Sensory Deprivation, Learning and Adjustment*. New York: Grune & Stratton, 1960.

Sherrill, C. *Adapted Physical Education and Recreation*. Iowa: Wm. C. Brown Co., 1977.

Wisher, Peter, "Therapeutic Values of Dance Education for the Deaf" in *Focus on Dance VII*, 3rd ed, Mason, K. C., ed. Reston, Virginia: AAHPER, 1974.

Kathleen Mason

Dance therapy can further the emotional and physical integration of the visually handicapped at various developmental stages. The blind infant and toddler need specific help in developing a concept of self and others and developing strong interpersonal relationships and unimpeded motor development (Fraiberg, 1971; Fraiberg, et al 1969). This is significant since children with obvious handicapping conditions risk developing maladaptive behaviors. Parental assistance may be vital if reactive behavior symptoms and unnecessary developmental delays are to be minimized and positive interaction maximized (Adelson and Fraiberg 1974; Chess and Hassibi 1978; Fraiberg and Friedman 1964).

Without continued encouragement and assistance, such as is offered by dance therapy, the young blind child is unable to experience the pleasure and mastery that movement normally brings to childhood. For older blind children and adults, dance therapy can help remediate restrictions in movement expression and can provide opportunities for socialization and communication. Dance therapy interactions can stimulate self-awareness and sensitivity to others. For the newly blinded individual contending with physical pain resulting from an inability to safely navigate the environment and psychological pain, fear, and anger, therapy is particularly important. Therapy may also help a sighted person faced with imminent blindness. In any of these situations, the intervention of a knowledgeable dance therapist may provide a catalyst to move the blind toward healthier functioning.

Basic Goals and Techniques

The goals of a dance therapist working with visually handicapped and nonhandicapped populations are comparable. No new theoretical base is needed to work with the blind. Needed is exploration and research into techniques to optimally facilitate therapeutic goals in view of specific visual limitations. Therapeutic modifications significant in work with visually handicapped individuals include: maximizing auditory, tactile, and kinesthetic stimuli; appropriately restricting the physical activity where physical conditions make it advisable; building the trust relationship fundamental to any therapeutic interaction.

The blind population is thought to diverge from the sighted in sensory and cognitive abilities, social and economic levels, moral values, movement skills, mental and physical health, and educational achievements. Yet persons with similar visual limitations may differ widely in adapting to their limitation. Cognizant of individual differences, the dance therapist must meet each person's level of functioning.

Developing a Trust Relationship

The dance therapist seeks to establish a trust relationship by reflecting back a person's movement qualities through the meaningful empathy of synchronous interaction. Vision is key and when this sensory modality is unavailable, additional aspects of nonverbal communication including spatial behaviors, facial expression, eye interaction and gesture become important in fostering a therapeutic relationship. Bodily contact and unified rhythmic interaction are elements of nonverbal communication that can be experienced directly by blind as well as by sighted individuals. Body contact can express affection, support, approval, and disapproval; moving rhythmically with another contributes to feelings of communion.

Verbal communication is also important to trust. The dance therapist's description of "the action" in a session informs and validates participants. Word choice by the therapist and participants indicates the closeness of group relationships. Semantics as well as paralinguistic aspects of language such as pacing, loudness, tonal quality, and extralinguistic sounds are important. A blind person's repeated sigh may alert others to feelings that that person is trying to convey. The members of one adult blind group spontaneously discovered that a unison sound of censure more effectively monitored one woman's cruel verbal attacks than did discussing them with her. Confronted with a consistent group response, she reduced the offending behavior without the defensive outbursts that followed direct confrontation.

Building a trust relationship requires protecting the blind person from physical injury resulting from the lack of vision. Maintaining optimal group size—relative to working space, the ages and visual limitations of members, the availability of assistants, and physical and/or emotional difficulties of group members—allows the leader to keep constant surveillance. If participants are unfamiliar with the room, or if furniture has been rearranged, they need to explore or "braille the room" as a blind counselor termed it. Blind children sometimes enjoy making a movement game of this. Holding onto waists, they follow the leader through the room space or do a simple folk dance that effectively defines the space. Children enjoy the challenge of locating changed or added furniture. Simplest and least time-consuming is to meet in a space least likely to be changed so that rather than accommodating to a new space, participants can explore interpersonal relations and feelings in the haven, comfort, and freedom of a predictable dance therapy space.

Important in establishing a trust relationship with blind participants is advising them of observers, as blind individuals often fear being viewed by others without knowing they are being watched. A sighted person, entering a new group, scrutinizes others' expressions to ascertain group acceptance and impact. Similarly, the verbalizations of a new member in a blind group, while appearing to be "incessant chatter," are a way of connecting with the group. These can be disconcerting to the therapist working with a group that has progressed to kinesthetic, tactile, and verbal exchanges relevant to feelings and thoughts in the movement experience context. This seems to be, however, a common step in group formation. It is also important to acknowledge when any member leaves the session.

Group trust grows as members share movement interaction. Often early work occurs individually or in twos, so a blind person's first attempts to move freely into space are eased by the accompaniment of another. Movement problems with a partner — such as moving with only fingertips touching — exploring balance, having a conversation with hands or feet, or discovering reciprocal movements within a rhythmic framework may begin a shared interaction. These experiences help group members discern emotional content in themes of meeting and parting, leading and following, supporting and being supported, and giving and receiving. Group

roles are explored as they move against, with, around and between other people and as they experience being far from, near to, and touching others (Preston 1963).

The circle, often used in dance therapy to encourage group cohesion, is effective with blind groups. A circle concept may be initially meaningless to those who lack sight, however, as eye contact often establishes the magic of the circle. Individuals in a circle may be aware only of having a person on either side of themselves. Instruments played by each person and passed around the circle, the whole group moving into the center and out to emphasize auditory voice changes on either side, and taking turns moving inside, outside, and around the circle to interact individually with each member, are ways the circle concept and one's part in it can be defined and internalized.

Using Other Sense Modalities

Contrary to popular belief, the blind, compared with sighted persons, do not have superior auditory or tactile senses (Chess and Hassibi 1978). Dance therapy experiences facilitate fuller use of alternative senses. Following directional voice or percussion instrument sounds, discriminating rhythmic movement patterns, and following tactile movement cues are possibilities for work in this area. Partially sighted children and adults are often less free in movement than completely blind individuals because they depend on residual vision and are not trained to use other sense modalities optimally (Chess and Hassibi 1978). Working with partially sighted individuals, it is helpful to have them experience movement part of the time with their eyes closed. This may be extremely frightening for some people at first; however, as they gradually develop auditory, tactile, proprioceptive, and kinesthetic senses, they may become less anxious about becoming totally helpless by losing their remaining sight. Working with individuals whose visual acuity fluctuates periodically requires particular sensitivity and understanding.

Learning to fully use alternative senses presents some problems. Young blind children often spontaneouly touch and smell objects and parts of other peoples' bodies. Although it is crucial that they develop their senses, they also need to learn social decorum. Adults who have become blind in adulthood generally are least comfortable using touch to explore and converse with others. Typically, propriety has more thoroughly conditioned them to control sensory exploration

Development of Movement Themes

Each group will develop and explore movement themes relevant to them. Some elementary school children spent part of each session for two weeks dealing with a theme common to blind children. It developed from group members singing "Row, Row, Row Your Boat" and moving out of the circle and back together again. One little boy "rowed" out of the circle, but instead of returning said, "My boat is lost." When we asked, "Do you want us to come find you?" he thought for awhile and replied that he did. The children all joined in the fantasy play and rowed their boats to find the lost one whom they embraced and helped home. This theme recurred daily with various resolutions. Once the children created one giant boat and rowed together. Another time, rocking their boats until they capsized, they swam to safety through shark-infested waters. During the final session, after being saved by the group, the boy who had instigated the theme volunteered, "You really didn't need to find me." Exploring this theme, children symbolically, yet actively, faced and gained some mastery over their fears.

Expression of Negative Feelings

Many blind individuals have difficulty expressing their anger toward those dear to them due to their dependence. Because the child needs the primary caretaker for emotional support and contact with the outside world, the child can't risk alienation. Especially for the adolescent faced with the developmental need to achieve independence, this presents a tremendous hurdle. Suppressing aggressive and sexual fantasies can have far-reaching consequences. The young person's phobic anxiety may project repressed impulses on objects in the environment. Some are arrested in uninsightful and repetitive play that contributes little to mastering the situation that prompted it (Wills 1968). Conversely, some blind people demonstrate no control over their aggression. They hurl verbal and physical abuse upon other people totally out of proportion to any actual grievance. Without differentiating between self and other, and with no control or object for aggressive acts, young people may be locked into self-abusive behavior. Constant acting-out, whether by child or adult, produces negative feedback from the environment and fixes the ego at an infantile level (Katan, 1964). Often punching clay, bouncing and throwing a ball or beating a drum releases anger. In one session, adults hurled their whole bodies against some thick mats hanging on a wall; pounding and punching they began verbally to connect with the sources of their pent-up frustrations.

The therapist can help group members identify and verbalize negative feelings. Beyond recognizing feelings, the group may serve as a socializing agent. The dance therapist can aid in the group process by interpreting and clarifying verbal and nonverbal feedback. With intrafamilial difficulties, dance therapy for the blind person's family may be helpful. Experience in relaxation and guided fantasy desensitizes sources of anxiety and promotes self-control. Through dance a person can channel negative affect into socially acceptable expression. Much of the work requires helping the blind discern cause and effect in both physical and social contexts. Only by experiencing the effect of their behavior on others can they begin to modify it to their own advantage (Chess and Hassibi 1978).

Movement Characteristics and Alignment

The exploration of body weight, centering, grounding, and static and dynamic positions can be important for blind individuals who have alignment difficulties. Exercises may be prescribed for the development of requisite muscle tonus, flexibility, and equilibrium. Equilibrium or balance without the important information to the brain that is offered by vision must be dependent upon vestibular input and proprioception. Difficulties in these areas are extremely detrimental to adequate functioning of the blind and may need to be treated with therapeutic methods to enhance sensory integration. Syndromes of sensorimotor dysfunction and a theoretical structure of activities to remediate difficulties are suggested in the writings of A. Jean Ayres (Ayres 1972).

Many blind individuals lack the "fighting efforts"[1] of suddenness and strength, expecially in conjunction with directness and free flow. Often coupled with this is shallow breathing (Weisbrod 1974) poor foot and knee articulation, and lower and upper trunk fusion — all causes of unstable grounding. Some blind individuals hold their bodies in constant vertical stress with extremely limited opening and closing in the horizontal plane or advancing and retreating in the sagittal plane. They walk leading alternately with the sides of the body.

---

[1]This term refers to the effort analysis of movement originated by Rudolph Laban. For a detailed explanation of Effort/Shape and supplementary concepts, see Bartenieff & Davis (1965), Dell (1970), Laban (1960, 1963), and White (1974).

Prevalent among many blind individuals, is restricted and/or inappropriate use of space. One elderly blind woman performed a punching movement as part of a group movement theme. Her punches used an "arc-like" rather than "spoke-like" path in space. She brought her arm straight to the front of her body, ending waist high, rather than bringing the bent arm up close to the body in front, and shooting it straight out in space. When she was taught how to punch effectively, she excitedly did the movement over and over again.

Sighted patients, and more frequently blind individuals, express fears connected with the space behind them. They are reluctant to move backward, to lean into that area, to fall, or even to gesture into that space.

Necessary remedial work, which enlarges movement vocabulary along with sense perceptions of movement, can give these individuals the bodily freedom to express ideas and emotions.

Blindisms

Blindisms—rocking, weaving the head from side to side, flipping hands before the eyes, and pressing the eyeballs — often become less frequent as children explore alternative movement. Satisfaction in more appropriate, less alienating emotional expression lessens the primitive movement habits yet in the initial stages of intervention, a ritualized movement such as rocking can help establish therapist/child interaction. As a relationship grows, the dance therapist may gradually introduce variations in time, energy, and space, thus transforming a blindism into shared patterns of varying complexity. How easily a blind child relinquishes isolating behavior in favor of human interaction indicates whether the behaviors are blindness-related or manifest psychiatric disorder (Chess and Hassibi 1978).

Language and Role Playing

A young child's language development helps inhibit movement responses. A child reaching for a forbidden bauble may say, "No touch, pretty" and stop a hand in midreach. Verbalization may also motivate the blind child. One little girl who was immobile and mute unless engaged in action by someone else was referred for dance therapy. The initial work helped her get in touch with her feelings and motivation and to overcome the fear of moving into the unknown. At first she was asked to make simple well supported decisions: "Should we move up together or down?" Later her words, "I

will walk to the slide," "I will take your hand," helped identify and move her intentions into action.

A blind child's early role play imitates sounds and words, first of his or her own role and later the roles of others. Since the child lacks visual recall of action, this play is largely verbal (Sandler and Wills 1965). A dance therapy session can help blind children extend role play into action by filling in gaps about the representational world and lessening motor inhibition. Active and verbal role play helps the child master feelings and differentiate make-believe from reality. Such play supports both the separation and integration of inner and outer stimuli.

Music in Dance Therapy Sessions

Because many blind people derive great pleasure from music, it can effectively promote free movement expression. An accompanist or a wide selection of recordings permits the therapist and group members to meet the mood and energy level of the moment. Often members will share personal record and tape collections. While this can help some persons become contributing members of the group, others use this to control and manipulate. Thus the therapist must always remain sensitive to the group's needs.

Body sounds — clapping, stamping, and finger snapping — also contribute to group cohesion. Spontaneous humming, chanting, and singing reinforce a variety of moods while having a powerful emotional impact upon participants. Prior to a holiday vacation, one group, sitting on the floor, ended a playful, high-energy dance interaction with hands joined. One person began to sing a Christmas song and others joined in. When the singing quieted, the mood had shifted and the participants began to recognize and deal with the isolation and depair many experienced during the "season to be jolly."

The Dance Therapist's Preparation

In addition to the skills and knowledge generally required of dance therapists, those who work with visually handicapped need to understand the developmental delays and problems resulting from lack of vision and the intervention processes which can facilitate optimal functioning at different developmental stages. They must understand a blind child's difficulties in forming a concept of self and others, establishing affective relatedness, and developing an adequate range of effort-shape movement qualities. They need to understand how the problems of the visually impaired differ from those of the totally blind and how any accompanying handicapping conditions can create additional limitations and stresses. The dance therapist needs to be able to differentiate behaviors directly resulting from or compensatory to blindness from those that indicate psychosis or autism. A dance therapist needs sensitivity in using touch and voice and selecting music.

Coming to terms with one's feelings associated with blindness is essential. Individual anxieties may revolve around issues such as one's own (1) dependency due to blindness or infirmity; (2) power or control over someone functioning less adequately; (3) rejection or anger resulting from the blinds' lack of "typical" nonverbal expressions of understanding and affiliation; (4) depression resulting from identification with the isolation and restricted initiative which many blind individuals experience.

References

Adelson, E., and Fraiberg, S. "Gross Motor Development in Infants Blind from Birth," *Child Development* 45: 114-126, 1974.

Ayers, Jean A. *Sensory Integration and Learning Disorders.* Los Angeles: Western Psychological Services, 1972.

Bartenieff, I. and Davis, M. "Effort-shape Analysis of Movement: The Unity of Function and Expression," New York, 1965. Reprinted in *Research Approaches to Movement and Personality.* New York: Arno Press 1972.

Chess, S. and Hassibi, M. *Principles and Practice of Child Psychiatry.* New York: Plenum Press, 1978.

Dell, C. *A Primer for Movement Description Using Effort-Shape and Supplementary Concepts.* New York: Dance Notation Bureau, 1970.

Fraiberg, S. "Intervention in Infancy: A Program for Blind Infants," *Journal of the American Academy of Child Psychiatry* 10:381-405, 1971.

Fraiberg, S., and Freedman, D. A. "Studies in the Ego Development of the Congenitally Blind Child." *The Psychoanalytic Study of the Child.* 19:113-169, 1964.

Fraiberg, S., Smith, M., and Adelson, E. "An Educational Program for Blind Infants," *Journal of Special Education* Vol. 3, No. 2, 1969. (121-139)

Katan, A. "Some Thoughts About the Role of Verbalization in Early Childhood," *The Psychoanalytic Study of the Child.* 16:184-188, 1964.

Laban, R., *The Mastery of Movement* 2nd rev. ed. Ullman, L. London: Macdonald & Evans, 1960.

Laban, R., and Lawrence, F. C. *Effort.* London: Macdonald & Evans, 1963.

Preston, V. *An Handbook for Modern Educational Dance.* London: Macdonald & Evans, 1963.

Sandler, A. M. and Wills, D. M. "Preliminary Notes on Play and Mastery in the Blind Child," *Journal of Child Psychotherapy I,* No. 3:7-19, 1965.

Weisbrod, J. "Body Movement Therapy and the Visually-Impaired Person," *Focus on Dance VII: Dance Therapy,* Mason, K., ed. Reston, Virginia: AAHPER, pp. 49-52, 1974.

Weitz, S., ed. "Paralanguage," *in, Nonverbal Communication: Readings with Commentary.* New York: Oxford Press, pp. 93-126, 1974.

White, E. "Effort-Shape: Its Importance to Dance Therapy and Movement Research." *Focus on Dance VII: Dance therapy,* Mason, K., ed. Reston, Virginia: AAHPER. pp. 33-37, 1974.

Wills, D. M. "Problems of Play and Mastery in the Blind Child." *British Journal of Medical Psychology,* 41(3):213-222, 1968.

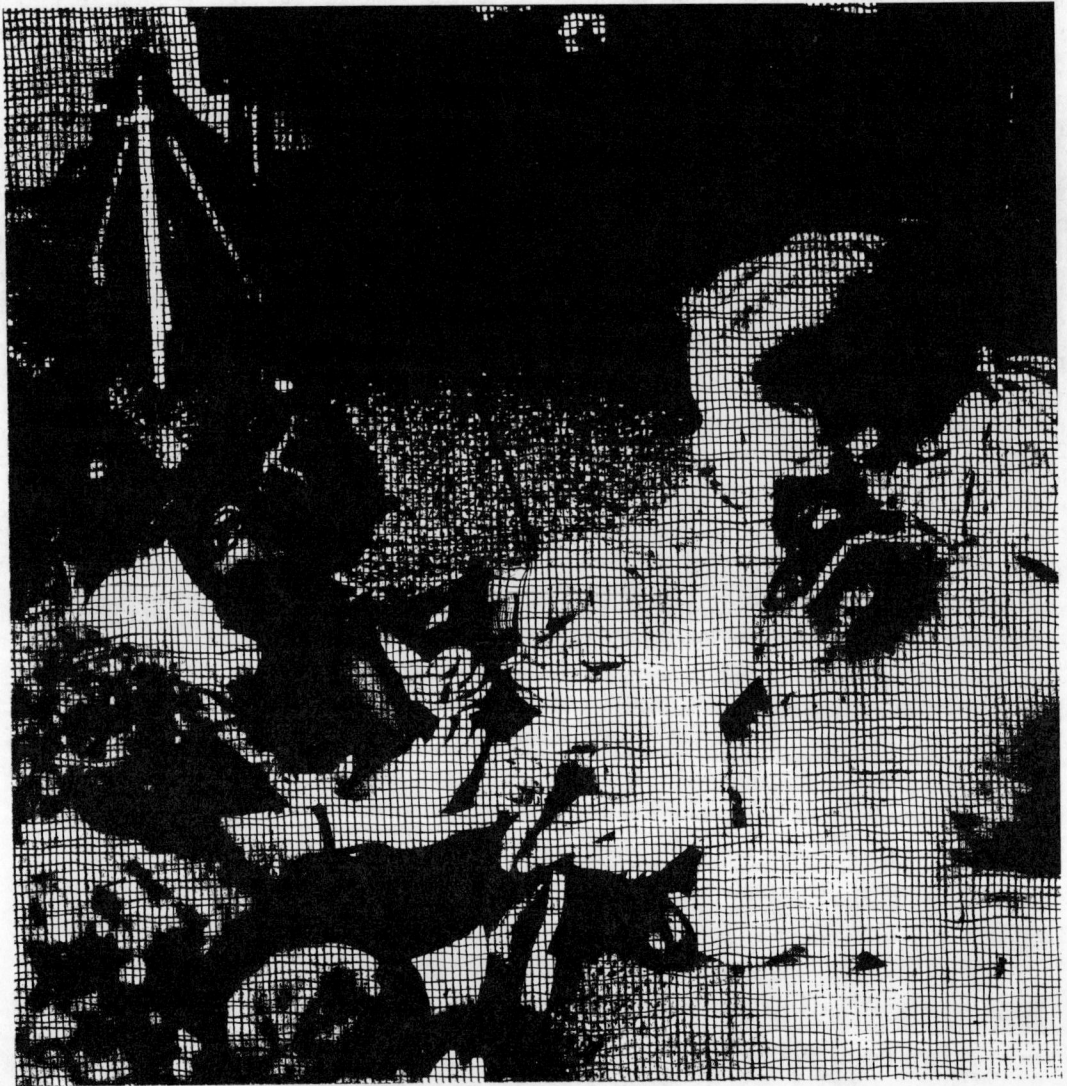

10 Dance Therapy as Treatment of Choice for the Emotionally Disturbed Learning Disabled Child

Marcia B. Leventhal

Dance Therapy and Mainstreaming

The intent of this chapter is to help educators and administrators, faced with choosing specialized services for handicapped children differentiate dance therapy from other body-oriented experiences, and to help dancers and physical educators learn to develop their skills toward dance therapy. The options have become particularly relevant since 1978 when including dance therapy as a related service under PL 94-192 permitted dance therapists to be hired under federally funded projects designed to improve the educational opportunities of handicapped children. In addition, dance therapists may be hired under the Comprehensive Employment and Training Act (CETA). While neither of these two policy-budget options preclude traditional dance therapy roles in special schools, psychiatric hospitals, mental health treatment centers and the like, it remains that recent years have seen a shift from dance therapy as only an *adjunctive* treatment to its use as a *primary* therapeutic modality.

To appreciate the virtues of dance therapy, rather than, creative dance, for example, as a treatment alternative for the emotionally or learning disabled child, one must understand the population to be served and fundamental differences between an educational and a therapeutic approach. The intent here is not to argue for one technique over another, but to show how dance therapy may be integrated into a total treatment scheme (social services, psychology, education). Two areas unique to the dance therapy model are the relationship of the leader to the population served and the methods used to develop basic force, time, space, and flow movement elements.

The Dance Movement Therapy Process

The wide theoretical base in dance-movement therapy is concerned with the development and subsequent integration of the total person. Its theory and methodology reflects the therapeutic powers (relationship, emotional development, symbolic manifestations of inner conflict), developmental movement, and movement expression. As a theory its technical applications may treat the area or areas of difficulty developmentally (using preverbal, dynamic skills) as well as the child's symptomatic manifestations of the emotional or behavioral disturbance.

In every activity of the child's day, his competency or lack of competency and experience is defined, expressed, and exposed through some aspect of movement: a gesture, a motion, or a change in energy flow. Research has shown a positive correlation between movement flexibility and range of choice, and the ability to think and to abstract (Hunt 1964). That children with problems are invariably inflexible in movement and therefore limited in their range of choice and ability to think and abstract are two considerations fundamental to developing dance-movement therapy programs

A Description of the Populations Being Served

The emotionally disturbed or learning disabled child, whether hyperactive with poorly defined body boundaries or hypoactive with rigid body boundaries has not developed an internal sense of time, space, or energy flow through which to receive and process spatial, temporal, and schematic cues from the environment. The following movement experiences all used within dance-movement therapy directly affect the child's perceptual motor and sensorimotor development and organization: (1) gravity or weight experiences, (2) body space (kinesphere) and environmental space (shapes, sequencing), (3) flow (interactional experiences within the dyadic therapist-child relationship). Often these children appear not to have developed a sense of their physical selves or of their center of gravity. By dealing with perceptual-motor or sensorimotor difficulties within the therapeutic relationship, positive behavior and prelearning changes occur rapidly. Dance therapy movement experiences build sequentially and developmentally from tactile-kinesthetic stimulation, to body part articulations, to weight and gravity experiences, to movement dynamics, to locomotion, and finally to expressive self-directed movement. Each component is a complete structure within itself but necessarily influences following areas, although a therapist may be working on two or three areas simultaneously.

Selected Results of Dance-movement Therapy Treatment

The child's heightened ability to learn and to become socialized results from dance-movement therapy and affects mainstreaming goals. Dance therapists work directly with sensorimotor and perceptual-motor development and integration to build or rebuild body image in its most primitive form through tactile and kinesthetic stimulation. The therapist's method in guiding the flow of the sessions positively affects the child's acquisition of pre-learning skills. Gratification delay, focusing, and the building of a positive self-concept, contributing to higher self-esteem and increased socialization are commonly manifested by children in treatment. How these results are developed and the methods which achieve them follow.

Dance therapy which deals with personal growth through body-mind interaction and expression, is founded upon a fundamental belief that movement expression reflects intra-psychic dynamics. The dance therapy model uses processes which unblock resistences to growth retained in a frozen musculature, rigid response or frozen postural patterns which necessarily limit feeling expression, perceptual reception, reality testing, or interpersonal relating. A fundamental belief holds that a change in movement expression results in a personality or behavior change; if range of feeling expression or perceptual reception is limited, then perception leading to reality testing and subsequent interpersonal relating will also be severely impeded.

Within the context of dance therapy, re-establishing a lost or distorted body image may strengthen self-concept at a preverbal level. Through experiences directed from flow or personal rhythmic expression, dance therapy may focus the hyperactive and calm the distraught and fearful, thus allowing growth to occur on a basic, body/developmental level. Movement is fundamental to all learning and dance therapy at its purest is a remedial, restructuring, "second chance" discipline.

Dance therapy is an integrative treatment process in which the therapist implements a developmental treatment plan which leads to a full trusting relationship with the child. Through the relationship alternative developmental paths for a child can be discovered. The therapist and child interact in space, with gestures, rhythms, and basic energy flow, and together create a language unique to their relationship, but universal in its results.

A Comparison of Dance Therapy to Creative Dance

Dance therapy and creative dance share basic tools: the moving body coping with force, time, space, and flow. But where creative dance encourages self-expression while building a technique and developing form, dance therapy encourages self-expression as a process between the therapist and the client/child to enhance emotional insight and interpretation through movement dialogue. The child's expression is viewed as a communication from the core of the self, rather than as pathologic or maladapted behavior. Thus it demands no performance or aesthetic standard, but rather encourages expression of those elements of motion which lead to motor generalization and motor skills. The dance therapist uses the child's behavioral or perceptual manifestations as thematic material for the therapeutic relationship which finally emerges as unencumbered spontaneous movement expression.

The Five-part Session: a Dance Therapy Model

Though each session is different and unique to the time, place and child, certain guidelines organize the development of a treatment plan. The model suggested here works toward an organic whole at each meeting: there is a beginning, a middle, and an ending. The five parts of each session include (1) warmup, (2) release, (3) theme, (4) centering, and (5) closure. The session may be viewed as a mini-life experience, reliable and easily repeatable as the child gains integrating capacity.

Children referred to dance therapy are fragmented in their perceptual development, exhibiting erratic and short attention. A dance therapy model which flows from beginning to end exposes the child to an external kinesthetic and perceptual model which ultimately serves as an internal foundation for more complex social and learning skills such as sequencing, generalizing, and closure.

During the warmup—which might last five minutes or five months, depending upon social, emotional, and motor development—a child is psychologically and kinesthetically prepared to be in the session. The warm-up begins where the child is, acknowledging the child's immediate presence by honoring body flow or expression. During the warm-up, the therapist attempts to release the tension set of the child, since residual tension or set patterns inhibit fully integrated motor expression.

During the middle section, thematic material expressed during the warm-up release and interpreted by the therapist, is explored with the child. During the thematic exploration, the therapist attempts to catalyze both the therapist/child relationship and the child's self-initiation. It is here that range exploration and development is encouraged.

The ending represents a "centering," a return to the here and now which encompasses two parts: anticipation of the next session and closure. This method offers the child a chance to say goodbye. Greeting and separation are experienced and learned. The session reflects life, as the child is offered the opportunity to experience completion, competency, and integration of the levels of relating and learning that occur in life.

The Development of the Therapist-Child Relationship

The child's overall behavioral functioning affects the therapist-child relation. A child's ability to attend within a formal session and to reorganize basic body image experiences determines how and when the therapist chooses to lead, follow, suggest, contrast, parallel, or mirror, all are styles of leading used by the dance therapist.

Because the therapist's training includes an ability to determine and view movement expression as reflective of intra-psychic dynamics, a child's patterns of expressive gestures or rituals are viewed as symbolic communications making sense within the child's ritualistic world. Within these communications, the therapist can often determine the child's level of fixation or regression. By relating through and/or planning motor interactions developed from the child's communication, the therapist facilitates completion of a child's social, emotional, or physical developmental level.

An understanding of ego development and object relating are essential, although only those essentials relative to treatment are included here. Briefly stated, the therapist encourages or stimulates through various movement experiences. These experiences express levels of organization through effort/shape and/or flow patterns.

The most primitive level of the child/therapist relationship is "autistic" communication; the child behaves ritualistically, unable to acknowledge the therapist apart from the ritual. Through patiently mirroring the child's movement rituals, the therapist builds toward a synchronous movement event in rhythm, flow, posture, or gesture. This event marks the emergence of the child to a symbio-tic orientation. At this level the therapist and child exchange supported, contained, and even merging body contact; holding and moving the child, the therapist helps develop kinesthetic experience. From this level, the therapist gradually helps a child progress to a parallel or mirroring relationship, finally—with verbal, visual, or imitative cues—helps the child move separately.

The therapist/child relationship, carefully nurtured, and the therapist's sensitivity to the child's movement expressions is crucial to dance therapy work. The therapist is sensitized to movement expression as it relates to the psychological, motor, and cognitive development of the child, since each of these is affected by the other in life, and problems in one area affect growth or integration in another. A child diagnosed as retarded or emotionally disturbed may in fact manifest a psychological trauma which has blocked perception, or the ability to integrate motor or cognitive skills. This complicated concern is beyond the thrust of this chapter, however, which is to show how dance therapy serves the development of the special child.

Over time a dance therapy session grows more perceptually complex and involves more risks by the child. Since expanding or altering ritual or rigid patterns involves lessening fear and developing trust, the child's sense of self must first be achieved. The therapist realizes how crucial are consistency, respect, and patience when working with the disturbed child.

Conclusion

To perceive, follow, and develop a child's movement cues, the dance therapist must have a broad movement-dance range free of dance stylization or personal idiosyncrasies. Along with group and individual leadership skills and expertise in psychology and psychodynamics, the therapist must remain free to move in and out of the often bizarre worlds of the disturbed child.

Movement time is self-discovery time. As a child discovers new movements effected by his own efforts, so do sense of self and well being grow proportionately. Dance therapy encourages fuller human functioning through communication between the inner and outer worlds.

As the emotionally disturbed youngster is able to let go of awkward body postures and attitudes, joy, release, and good feelings become more frequent. As a child gains control of the most basic self, the body, as a more flexible range of movement using force, time, and space create a new world of ease, so do contacts with the outside world become more available and appropriate. Techniques, methods and lessons are not inherent to dance therapy, but range development, use and encouragement of non-verbal communication, and full acceptance of the child's pre-verbal symbols are the core of the dance therapy model.

References

Dell, Cecily. *A Primer for Movement Description*. New York: Dance Notation Bureau, 1970.

Hunt, Valerie. "Movement Behavior: A Model for Action," in *Quest, Monograph II*. Tucson, Arizona: NAPECW and NCPEAM, Spring, 1964.

Leventhal, Marcia B. "Movement Therapy with Minimal Brain Dysfunction Children," in Mason, Kathleen, ed. *Dance Therapy: Focus on Dance VII*. Reston, Virginia: AAHPER, 1974. pp. 42-48.

—————————. "Structure in Dance Therapy; a Model for Personality Integration," in Rowe, Patricia and Stodelle, Ernestine, eds. *Dance Research Collage, Annual X*. New York: Congress on Research in Dance, CORD 1979.

Mahler, Margaret, Pine, Fred and Bergman, Anni. *The Psychological Birth of the Human Infant*. New York: Basic Books, Inc., 1975.

11 Procession: Developmental Dance with Disabled People

Gertrude Blanchard and Dan Cieloha

*pro • ces • sion: n. (< L < pro-forward + cedere to go)
a group of people or things moving forward in an orderly
sequence.*

Whether you think of a procession as a parade, or
the opening of a church service, or the events of
history, or the movement of the planets, you think
of *order* and *moving forward*. The teaching of dance
to disabled people often is not orderly, often does
not move forward, rarely is developmental. Our
goals as educators should underline teaching more
than exposing, training more than entertaining,
learning more than experiencing. To do this we
must concentrate on simple and logical patterns of
growth.

All of us cannot be Joan Sutherlands, Willie
Mayses, Martha Grahams, Bruce Jenners, Wilma
Rudolphs, or Helen Kellers, but the process which
trained their talent is open to everyone. Few wish or
are able to achieve stardom, for it necessitates a
narrow life focus. For people with disabilities the
goal is often as demanding as that of any famous
achiever. What they win, however, is a different
distinction: the ability to live independently.

Let us suppose that you have a disabled child. If
you feel that you cannot imagine realistically, spend
a day in a wheel chair, on crutches, or wearing a
blindfold. You would want for your child all the
competencies that would enable him to live an independent life: communication, independent
movement, everyday skills, the ability to think and
feel, the strength and wisdom to accept the handicap and still find life worthwhile. You would want
any educator who was working with your child to
be supportive of many of his needs, not movement
alone.

"The Process" is the subject of this paper, and a
term which will be used frequently in the following
pages. Briefly, it is a developmentally oriented system for teaching movement and movement-related
vocabulary, designed to provide training in physical, mental, and social/emotional skills. Specifically
it presents dance at the learning level, and provides
a solid base from which each individual can explore

dance as a form of personal communication and
expression.

There are many systems for teaching dance, but
the one offered here (1) has been tested over a
period of many years with physically, mentally,
and neurologically disabled people; (2) offers little
opportunity for imitation, thus stimulating both
thinking and creativity; (3) stresses basic vocabulary rather than esoteric dance terms; and (4) focus-
ses on measurable growth rather than experiences.

The Process makes dance possible for everyone.
Based on our experience both the objectives and the
methods are adaptable to all individuals regardless
of disability, although its impact and effectiveness
are often considerably less visible among physically
and mentally low-functioning people. To date we
have not devised a satisfactory measure to determine whether this less visible effectiveness is related directly to the limitations of the curriculum, or
whether it can be attributed to the lack of a common
system of communication between the teacher and
the learner. However, in our work with children
and adults who are identified as mentally retarded,
mentally ill, emotionally, physically, and learning
disabled, and visually and hearing impaired, we
have regularly observed positive results in response
to the curriculum.

Two points need to be borne in mind. (1) The
Process is not primarily therapeutic. Therapeutic
modalities may move the individual toward realizing an ideal in one specific way. This can be very
helpful in learning to walk in a way that is a reliable,
long-term means of ambulation. The ideal in The
Process, however, can best be realized in the very
multiplicity of responses that the concept of walking may evoke. Steve (spina bifida) can walk on his
hands; Alicia (cerebral palsy) can do a hip walk.
Both can physically demonstrate their understanding of the shifting of body weight from one part to
another, resulting in movement in any direction.
The Process encourages the individual to retain responsibility, to listen, to think, and to self-actualize
his response. The implications of this manner of

47

teaching/learning with disabled people are especially significant. In the therapuetic sense, Steve must learn to use crutches; Alicia must adapt to leg braces. In the dance sense, each uniquely solved the problem through thinking. (2) Often much of a disabled person's life is spent in therapy directed to a particular body part or function. The Process does not ignore this need, but strives to teach the whole person, the sum of the affective, the cognitive and the physical. To experience wholeness is a rare opportunity for most disabled people.

The purpose of The Process is teaching to and with the whole person, even though we analyze our objectives in three categories. The learner is provided (1) physically, with gross and fine motor coordinations in isolation and combination, using various perceptual faculties: visual, auditory, tactual; (2) cognitively, with a structure for learning that requires listening, thinking, remembering, and a demonstrable motor response to cognitive input; (3) affectively, with practice in appreciation, kindness, cooperation, decision making, responsibility, and courtesy: the oil for the machinery of human relations. The objectives cannot be viewed, nor can they be accomplished, in isolation. There is a simultaneity that is at once the excitement as well as the success of The Process. It is imperative, too, that the person self-actualize these objectives. If they come from outside his experiene, their value is diminished.

The methods used in teaching movement developmentally have familiar names.

1. Assessment and Analysis
   A. Assess what is known
   B. Select a concept
   C. Analyze the concept
2. Construct a developmental sequence: lesson plan
3. Lesson presentation
4. Evaluation.

What may not be so familiar to the dance educator is the detail necessary to making the lesson developmental.

Assessment/analysis helps you to decide where to begin. If you are meeting the group or individual for the first time, a talk with the therapist, classroom teacher, psychologist, and other specialists will provide answers to many questions. What are the learner's physical, mental, and emotional limitations and strengths? What words does he understand? Can he communicate? What behavior is he able to control? What is his attention span? What is his attitude? Are there things you must not do? At approximately what grade level does he function?

Be sure to make friends with the learner and give him a chance to get used to you. Let him express, verbally or otherwise, his ideas and feelings.

The focus of movement learning in The Process is to teach and reinforce not only dance concepts, but also words from the Dolch List (Dolch 1942) and Boehm Test (Boehm 1971), which can be demonstrated and understood using the learner's own body.

To do this you must analyze and define the components of the concept you have chosen. What movement, knowledge, and behavior is required? Can you teach it with known words? What are the unknowns you must teach? Can you organize the elements from simple to complex, building logically?

Once you have assessed and analyzed, chosen your concept, and found its components, you are ready to construct a developmental sequence which will be your lesson plan. It should include not only the specifics of the concept, but also the fringe benefits. If it is a first lesson, how will you introduce yourself and explain what you are going to do? How will you develop friendliness and trust? Will you do a review of any kind? Is thinking, listening, and remembering required? What decisions does the learner have to make? What interactions will there be with you or others? What will you do if the learner does not respond appropriately?

You are now ready to plan your presentation. Probably the most important part of your teaching will be the questions you ask, not the answers you give. Your questions must be so skillful and phrased so simply that the learner can discover the answers. Where there is verbal communication, you will plan what the learner will say and do, read and do. You will plan to demonstrate only when the simplest verbal instruction is not understood, but you will continue the simple, verbal instruction while demonstrating. You will manipulate where necessary and acceptable. Your plan will include time for praise and approval, time to call attention to good efforts, thinking, and interaction. You will decide how to soothe the fears of one, stimulate the actions of another, demand of the lazy; and, if the excitement runs too high, plan a cool down of body, mind and emotions before the end of the lesson. Throughout the teaching you will adhere religiously to your carefully thought out lesson plan, making only such changes as moving at a slower pace, exploring more thoroughly, backing up more than moving speedily. Your plan will, however, include alternative ideas, motivations, gimmicks, and so on, which you will use if the learner does not respond to your initial approach, but you will not

1		2		3
Assess learner's knowledge and abilities	→	Select appropriate concept for instruction	→	Analyze concept

6		5		4
Evaluation of learner, teacher, and lesson.	←	Lesson presentation.	←	Construct teaching sequence (lesson plus).

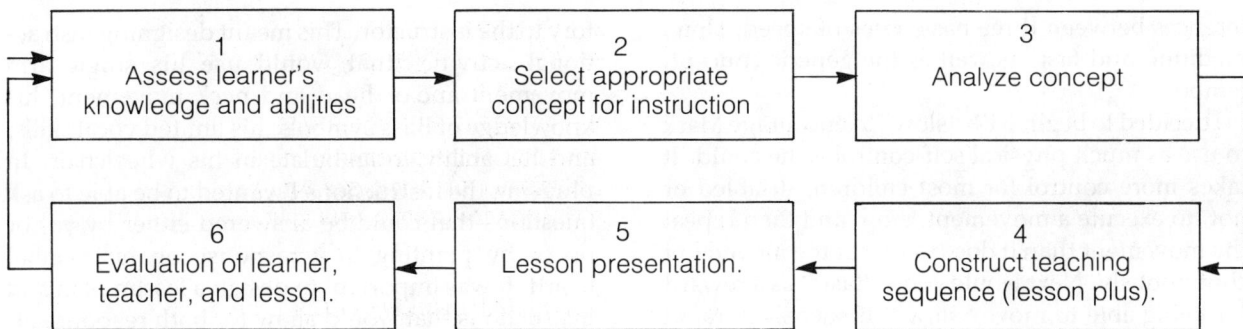

introduce unrelated materials or wander off into flights of creativity. At the end your plan will have moved the learner from A to B, possibly to C. You will know that in your next lesson you can assume A and B, and possibly C, with review, and proceed to the next developmental step.

Evaluation goes on concurrently with teaching as well as in those lonely, self-analytical times after class. You will be training your eye to make continuing perceptive observations of the learner's performance. From this you will make corrections and suggestions, for responses, verbally and physically, are not always worthy of the learner's ability. To test learning, you will eliminate the opportunity for limitation, and see if the class or individual can solve the problem, give the definition, or move in the correct manner. The evaluation results will show in your next lesson plan.

The model above charts the sequence for preparation and presentation of The Process. The discussion of methods may seem unnecessarily detailed, but every item must be planned if the stated physical, cognitive, and social-emotional goals are to be achieved. If you are going to make development happen, you cannot "wing it."

How these methods are used, with specific concepts and disabilities is described in the ensuing three examples. (You might like to construct a lesson plan of your own, based on The Process description, and then check it against one of ours.) Several points need to be emphasized. (1) Dance — which may be enjoyable, beautiful, communicative — is movement which is important to the dancer. (2) It cannot be assumed that many basic words are understood. (3) Understanding may be clear even though performance may not be precise. (4) To move within the meaning of a concept takes training, and often thinking. (5) The Process is applicable to any handicap, and the examples include physical, mental, and emotional disabilities.

Example 1

Mark is a seven year old boy with cerebral palsy. It is a congenital condition that does allow for limited range of motion in his right arm, some voluntary control of his torso, neck, and head. He has little control over his over extremities. His vocal abilities are limited to forming some vowel and consonant sounds, but he cannot yet form intelligible polysyllabic words. He has recently begun instruction in Bliss symbolics (Blissymbolics Communication Foundation). This alternative form of written communication reduces an entire word to a single symbol. For example, water is represented by the symbol ∿. For most activities Mark is in a wheelchair or lying on the floor. He orients well to surrounding space. In fourteen previous half-hour individual sessions Mark demonstrated his understanding of all concepts presented, both initially and in subsequent sessions.

Mark can move forward and backward for short distances and can turn his wheelchair. What would be an appropriate next step for anyone with these abilities? What could be progressive, challenging but not impossible, and eventually incorporated into a variety of movements and movement sequences? We concluded that tempo (slow, medium, and fast) would be an appropriate next concept. In the instructional design we also planned to include the following words that Mark already knew: big, little, near, far, body part names, touch, begin (go), stop, same, different, opposite, between, other, more, and less.

In analyzing the concept and its physical manifestations, it seemed that tempo, as a concept involving time and space, could be understood by Mark if he could hear, see, or feel a sound, movement, or tactile stimulus repeated at specific intervals. It was important to develop movement activities that would allow Mark to feel and understand the differences between three basic rates of speed, slow, medium, and fast, as well as the generic concept, tempo.

I decided to begin with "slow" to encourage Mark to use as much physical self-control as he could. It takes more control for most children, disabled or not, to execute a movement, stop, and then repeat the movement than it does to repeat the movement continuously. Next would come "fast," as a reward for being able to move "slow." If success at rapid repetitive movements could be achieved, we would then begin to explore and define that which was neither slow nor fast: medium.

Teaching this concept with Mark's body as the primary learning tool would involve adaptations to meet his physical limitations. By looking for what Mark could do, a strategy for presentation was devised that seemed realizable for Mark and satisfac-

tory to the instructor. This meant designing instructional activities that would use his single arm movement and/or head and neck movement, his knowledge of Bliss symbols, his limited vocal skills, and his ability to ambulate in his wheelchair. In phrasing the instructions I wanted to be able to ask questions that could be answered either by yes or no or by pointing to a response on his symbol board. It was important to design a lesson plan and instructions that would allow for both response alternatives. One objective was to integrate the use of the symbol board into the lesson when his having to stop and point at it would not interfere with the general flow of his movement experience. In addition, there needed to be opportunities for verbal and body communication.

The lesson plan and sample of verbal instructions used with Mark follow:

LESSON PLAN

1. Introduction. Examples of slow to fast continuum.
   a. rocket launch
   b. runner in football
   c. race car start
   d. moving in wheelchair

2. Slow—using:
   near
   far
   body parts
   touch

3. Slow—using:
   body parts
   touch
   big
   more
   other

VERBAL INSTRUCTIONS

1b. When the receiver catches the ball, how does he begin to run. Slow or fast?
1d. When you begin to go forward in your wheelchair are you going fast or slow?
When we talk about how fast or slow something goes, we're talking about tempo. Tempo is how fast or slow anything moves, sounds, or feels.

2. Move your hand as far from your head as you can. Good. Now, can you get your hand to come so near your head that you could touch it? Great. Try it again. Hand far, hand near. Hand far, hand near. Hey, that's really fine. See if you can make your hand go far or near every time you hear the sound of the drum. Is that like beginning to move in your chairs? Yes. It's slow. It's not fast. Let's do it once more. Hand near, slow. Hand far, slow. Slow, slow, slow, slow.

3. Mark, can you find a way to make your ear touch your shoulder? How about the other ear touching the other shoulder? Try bringing your ear even more near. Can you make it touch your shoulder? When I touch your other shoulder bring your other ear near to the shoulder I'm touching. Good. Now, every time I touch a shoulder move your head so that one ear is near to the shoulder I touch. That's it; keep going.

Let's rest for a minute. You're really doing a good job. When you move your head from one shoulder to the other what kind of movement is it? Is it big or little? Right. It's about the biggest movement your head can make. When you move big can you move fast? Well, try doing it again. See if you can tell. You're right, it's pretty slow, it's not fast at all. Here watch me do it. Is my head moving slow or fast?

LESSON PLAN	VERBAL INSTRUCTIONS

LESSON PLAN

4. Fast — using:
   big
   little
   body parts
   same
   different

5. Fast — using:
   near
   far
   body parts
   same
   different

6. a. Tempo
   b. fast
   c. slow
   using:
   body parts

7. Reinforce
   tempo
   fast
   slow
   Introduce
   between
   medium

8. Reinforce all three tempo
   components
   slow
   medium
   fast

VERBAL INSTRUCTIONS

4. Mark, when you tell me 'no' with your head, is that a big movement? Do your ears move all the way to your shoulder? Try it. Exactly. Your head makes just a little movement. Try it again. Does it take a lot of time to say 'no' with your head? Right again. It takes just a little time to make a little movement. Here Mark, look in the mirror. Try saying no with your head again. Is your head moving slowly? Look carefully. It's not the same, it's not big like when ears go all the way to shoulders. It's different. Right. It's just a little movement. It's fast. Fast. Try moving your head as fast as the drum sounds.

5. Now, when you hear the drum the first time, touch your head. When you hear it again move your hand far from your head. Next drum sound touch your head again. Next sound, hand far from head. 1, 2, ready, go. Well, can you let your hand go far from your head and still move as fast as the drum sounds? No? You're right. Your hand has to stay near your head to move it fast. Try it again with the drum. That's the way — fast, fast, fast, fast, fast.

6a. Mark, that new word for how fast or slow something goes, what letter does it begin with? Right, 't'. The word's tempo. Tempo.

6b. This time when you hear the fast tempo on the drum move some part of your body fast. 1, 2, ready, go. OK, your hand moving fast to touch your head, that's fine. Can you find another way? Good, one finger can move very fast.

6c. Listen to this slow tempo. Can you move some part of your body slowly? Good, your mouth can move as slowly as the tempo. Stay right with it. Don't go faster. Here, see if you can beat a slow tempo on the drum. All right Mark?

7. Mark, keep the drum on your lap. Play the drum at a fast tempo. Fine. Now try a slow tempo like you did before. Good. Can you play the drum at a tempo that's not fast and not slow? Yes, that tempo's between slow and fast. Keep it going. That's me-di-um, me-di-um, me-di-um. Keep going. Me-di-um, me-di-um. Don't let it get fast. Good. And stop. When the tempo isn't fast and isn't slow, when it's between slow and fast it's me-di-um. Medium. Here, I'll take the drum.

8. I'm going to play the drum at one tempo. Point to the correct word on your symbol board for that tempo. Fine, Mark. Here's another one. See if you can tell what this one is.

This time you decide how you want to move when you hear the drum. You can make your wheelchair move at a fast tempo. Or, you can move your arm at a medium tempo, or you might move your head slowly when you hear a slow tempo. Here, let's try some.

At the session's conclusion I felt that we had met the objective set when designing the lesson plan. A new concept word, tempo, had been introduced to Mark, its three component elements, slow, medium, and fast had been reinforced in tactile, kinesthetic, and cognitive ways, and a large number of previously learned concept words were employed within the verbal instructions.

Modes of communication and their appropriateness to the specific activity or task were a continuing source of concern throughout the session. Mark had been working in Bliss symbols for only six weeks when this session took place. I was still experimenting with ways to use this alternative communication system most effectively. While the basic criterion for using the symbol board was to see whether or not it would interrupt the flow of Mark's movement, in actuality I found myself, in the interest of time, accepting Mark's nod or an uttered sound as sufficient response to a question. By asking some questions that merely required a yes or no response, I created a situation where I was providing the concept words for Mark, (Is this fast?) rather than encouraging him to seek out the appropriate symbol word on his board, (What tempo is this?). A better balance could have been struck between the two styles of questioning.

As a result of the session's work I became more aware of the need to consciously construct questions, activities and, most of all, time frames that would encourage Mark to fully use both communi-cation systems and to incorporate them into the activity with increasing comfort.

Example 2

The learners are a class of twelve visually impaired, nine and ten year old boys and girls, functioning academically at a third grade level. Some have been blind from birth, some have lost their sight through injury, some are partially sighted. All are otherwise physically and mentally normal. They have the usual insecurities and fears: of being alone in space; of bumping, falling, stumbling into the unknown. None is afraid to be touched; all have good attention. They are a group fairly well adjusted to their handicaps, with personality manifestations typical of their ages. From previous lessons or other sources, they can name and identify body parts. They understand the meanings of the following words: front, side, level, bend/stretch, fast, slow, large, small, big, little, apart, together, movement, close, distance, between, high, different, size, partners. Based on their abilities and what they know, we chose for their next developmental step the concept of *tempo*.

We defined tempo as the rate or measure of speed at which something moves or sounds, but we decided to let the students find their own definition. The components we chose were slow, fast, and medium. We hoped to lead the students to the discovery of the relationship between tempo and size. This is a forty-five minute lesson.

LESSON PLAN	LESSON PRESENTATION
(I must be sure to run through this with my eyes closed, using the exact words of the presentation, thinking of what I am hearing.)	(I must keep in mind that to the blind I am a radio, not a TV; that the use of the word "see" and variations is all right.)
1. Hand claps, fast, sitting level	1. Can you hold the palms of your hands so close together that you could just feel a piece of paper between them? Can you clap your hands, keeping them close to each other? Try to do it faster.
2. Hands claps, slow	2. Hold your hands as far apart as you can. Now see if you can clap slowly, because you have a great big distance between your hands.
3. Hand claps, medium	3. Can you hold your hands as far apart as your shoulders? Clap them from this distance. That is a medium clap, between fast and slow.
4. Respond to varied slow, fast, medium drum beats and clapping	4. Listen to the drum, and see if you can clap your hands at whatever speed the drum is beating, using small/fast, big/slow, and medium size claps.

LESSON PLAN	LESSON PRESENTATION

5. Foot claps, fast, slow, medium

5. Can you clap the soles of your feet together? That's hard, isn't it? Hold them as close together as you did your hands when you clapped fast, and clap them as fast as you can. Now make the biggest movement you can with your legs, and clap slowly. Now try medium, between fast and slow.

6. Standing level; walk/run in place, fast

6. Can you lift one foot off the floor just far enough so that I could slip a piece of paper under it? Try it with the other foot. Now run, in place, as fast as you can, keeping your feet very close to the floor.

7. Walk/run, slow

7. Lift your foot as high as you can, do a very slow walk right in place.

8. Walk/run, medium

8. Lift your foot just as high as your knee, and do a medium walk.

9. Respond to varied slow, medium, fast drum beats and walk/run

9. Listen to the drum, and see if you can make your feet walk/run at whatever speed the drum is beating.

10. Claps with sounds, fast, slow, medium; standing level

10. Let's do fast claps again, standing this time, and see if you can make voice sounds go as fast as your hands. What is the shortest, fastest sound you can make? I hear some good ones that you could do very fast. If you are not sure, think of the sound of water dripping, or a pencil tapping. Now find a long, slow sound that would go with slow claps; now a medium sound that would go with medium claps.

11. Respond to varied slow, fast, medium drum beats.

11. Listen to the drum, and see if you can clap and make your sounds at whatever speed the drum is beating.

12. Sitting level, synonyms

12. Can you think of other words that mean fast? (quick, speedy, swift) slow? (creep, crawl, drag, like a snail) medium? That's a hard one. What about in the "middle" or "intermediate"? Do you know those words? "In between" — that's a good one.

13. Tempo

13. We have been making movements and sounds at different speeds — fast, slow, medium. The fastness, slowness, or mediumness with which one moves or speaks has a special name: tempo. Will you say the word? Tempo. Say it again. Tempo. You may know about music, and may have heard the word used in playing and singing. There it is how fast, slow, or medium you play or sing. But it is also used to tell about the speed with which you move. What was the new word? Tempo. Right.

14. Size and tempo

14. Did anyone notice any difference in the size of our movements? Were the fast movements big or little? Slow movements large or small? Medium movements? Could you make a big, fast movement? Yes, you could, but it wouldn't be as fast as the little, fast movement. Could you make a little, slow movement? Yes, but what? Right! It wouldn't be as slow as the big slow movement. It's helpful to remember that big is usually slow, little is usually fast, and medium is between the two.

LESSON PLAN	LESSON PRESENTATION
15. The plural of tempo: tempi Other examples	15. When we speak of more than one rate of movement, or speed, or the plural of tempo, it is called "tempi." Will you say it? Tempi. Right! Can you think of other examples of tempi? Not claps, or voice sounds, or walk/run. (Little Engine That Could; swinging high, medium, low; jumping rope; different sized bells — jingle, school, church; hair brushing — short, medium, long; bouncing balls.)
16. Bouncing balls with varied tempi	16. Listen to the sound of the bouncing ball, and tell me whether you think it is going slow, medium, or fast. Which bounces are big? little? medium?
17. Those who want to try working with balls	17. Would some of you like to try to bounce a ball? Raise your hand if you want to try, and I'll bring you a ball. Stay on the sitting level, but spread your legs apart so that you can do the bounces between your legs. I am going to come to each of you and let you feel my hand while I bounce fast. Then you can try it while I move on to someone else. Don't worry if the ball hits your leg and rolls away. I'll get it and bring it back to you. Use both hands and you will find it easier. See how fast you can bounce the ball with very small movements. If you want to, you can get on knee level, and try some medium bounces. Keep the ball close to your body and be gentle. Those who want to may try standing level and slow bounces. Don't let the ball go any higher than your chin and it will be easier to know where it is.
18. Bend/stretch: fingers, torso, whole body	18. Let's put the balls away for today, and sit down again. Can you stretch your fingers so that they are very straight and far apart? So that I could take a pencil and draw around each finger and thumb and make a picture of your hand? Now bend your fingers so that they make a fist; and stretch them again; and bend — stretch, bend-stretch. See how fast you can bend/stretch your fingers. Try to stay with the drum. Get on the knee level, and bend your torso forward, down toward the floor; then stretch it tall, making your head reach for the ceiling. Do it again, medium speed, medium size. On the standing level, bend your whole body, then reach for the ceiling, up on your toes if you can. Do it again, a big, slow bend, a big, slow stretch.
19. Respond to slow, fast, medium drum, changing levels and body parts	19. Listen to the drum. If it beats fast, you will do finger bend/stretches on the sitting level; if it beats medium, you will do torso bend/stretches on the knee level; if it beats slowly, you will do whole body bend/stretches on the standing level. Do you understand? Let's try it. What good listening and thinking. You did a beautiful job.
20. Combining tempi and clapping, walk/runs, on standing level	20. Let's all get on the standing level and remember how we did tempi with claps and walk/runs. We're going to try to do two different tempi with two different movements, and do them both at the same time. I will not be beating the drum. You will choose your own fast, medium, slow. Show me fast claps. Keep clapping fast and see if you can make your feet go with big, slow steps in place. Good. Now try big, slow claps, with little fast feet. Here's another one: medium feet (as high as your knees) and fast hands. Can you think of a combination we haven't tried? Good for you. Fast hands, fast feet; medium hands, slow feet; slow hands, slow feet; medium hands, medium feet.

LESSON PLAN	LESSON PRESENTATION
21. Bend/stretch tempi, with body parts but all on standing level.	21. Let's try the same thing with bend/stretch, but stay on the standing level all of the time. Can you do a fast finger bend/stretch at the same time you are doing a slow body bend/stretch? How about a medium torso bend/stretch with a fast finger bend/stretch? Congratulations! That was great!
22. With partners, face to face, holding hands; with drum; at the end try 2 slow, 4 medium, 8 fast, but do not teach the phrasing.	22. I'll help you get partners, and you'll stand face to face holding both of your partner's hands. It's so nice to see that all of you are friends and like being partners with anyone in the class. That's really very grown up. The first thing you are going to do, while holding hands, is to move your arms as far apart as they were when you did slow claps. You will have to stand quite close to each other. Try moving your arms apart/together slowly. Good! Remember medium? as far apart as your shoulders? Try apart/together, medium. Fast was very close. Try moving apart/together fast. Now you have practiced all the tempi, try staying with the drum beat.
23. Tempi, body parts, side by side, standing level, near arms clasped or hooked, with drum; end with 2 slow, 4 medium, 8 fast, but do not teach the phrasing.	23. Now stand side by side with your partner and join your near arms in a comfortable way. Try whole body, slow, bend/stretched together; now torso bend/stretches, medium, finger bend/stretches, fast. Now see if you can do all three staying with the beat of the drum.
24. Combine face to face and side by side tempi, using arms and body parts, standing level, with drum; continue as long as they are enjoying it.	24. We're going to put the face to face and side by side movements together, and we'll see how good your memories are. I will call out "face to face" or "side by side", slow, medium, or fast. You will get into the correct position, and use your arms and hands, or your fingers, torso, or whole body to do what is right for the position and tempo I name. Do you understand? Here we go! Everybody side by side, slow; face to face, slow; face to face, medium; side by side fast; side by side medium; face to face, fast; etc. etc. etc.
25. Checking	25. That was a good job. I liked the way you were helping each other, and the way some of you were laughing and giggling while you were moving. Now let's sit down and talk a bit. Raise your hand if you can tell me what tempo means? (It's how fast or slow or medium you move—or sing—or drive a car—or a train, etc.) Good! Who can tell me the meaning of the word "medium"? (It's between fast and slow, or big and little; or between opposites.) Tell me what you mean by "between opposites." (Like between tall and short is medium, or between fat and skinny, or between good and bad, I guess.) That's very good thinking. What can you tell me about size and tempo? (Big things are usually slow moving; little things usually go fast—like elephants and ants.) That's a good way to say it: "like elephants and ants."
26. Cool down	26. Everyone on the lowest level; stretch your whole body until it's as big as you can make it on the floor; curl up until you're as small as you can make yourself; stretch again, bend again; stretch again and stay stretched, but relax, go limp with your arms, your neck, your legs, your back. Let your whole body be limp and relaxed, and just think about breathing, slowly. Breathe as slowly as your arms moved apart and together; as slowly as your whole body moved doing bend/stretch. When you feel relaxed and rested, get up, come to me, and we'll see how many of you can find your own shoes and socks.

Both the learning and the teaching need to be evaluated.

The class had a tightness of movement throughout, partially due to their being in a strange room. A longer time could have been spent on each problem, but we moved on while they were still enjoying. They had good attention and memory, excellent effort, quite good balance. They handled the vocabulary well, supplied good definitions of tempo and medium, and satisfactory answers to questions. They would have enjoyed more time with balls, but need a lesson on ball handling unrelated to tempo. Overall, verbal responses were better than physical responses.

More time should have been spent on body preparation and familiarizing the class with the new space. It was difficult to praise much of the movement because it was not as good as they could do, and I did not want to set low standards of approval. The lesson progression was good, and there was good rapport between the class and me. Although I used the 2/4/8 drum beat, I did not teach phrasing. I wanted the class to get used to hearing a set phrasing, as well as responding to random phrasing. Teaching some phrasing should probably be the next step, followed by the class developing some simple combinations and phrases of their own. I need to work on "limp" in the cool down. I did not teach it, and their understanding was not sufficient to make their performance beneficial.

Example 3

Nora is a forty-seven year old woman who was committed to a state mental institution when she was twenty. Two years ago she was released from that institution and placed in a board and care home near the community where she grew up. Nora's doctor has prescribed daily medication intended to lessen the degree of mind change she usually experiences in the course of a day.

Four days each week she participates in a day program at a local community center. On one of those days I work with Nora on an individual basis. In these sessions her behavior can best be described as erratic. If she has taken her medication she may be very attentive to our work or she may be listless and apathetic. On the other hand, when she has not taken the medication she is usually uncooperative, suspicious, and hostile.

When I first saw Nora her shoulders were contracted forward, head bowed, back rounded and arms alternately drawn in toward the center of her body or crossed in front of her. She walked with a slow, shuffling gait. After talking with others who worked with Nora and observing her as she interacted with others at the Center, it seemed that her physical presentation was not the result of any specific physical disability but seemed instead to be a handicap acquired through years of relative inactivity while institutionalized. She had good fine motor skills and enjoyed sewing, stitchery, and other handicrafts.

Her usage and apparent understanding of words was as unpredictable as many of her other behaviors. Often she would communicate in complete "adult" sentences. She could also follow complex verbal instructions. There were times, however, when her communication would consist of monosyllables, grunts or whines, and she would seem not to comprehend the simplest of verbal instructions. We also felt that these behaviors might also be related to Nora's long-term institutionalization.

The goal in working with Nora was to develop movement and dance-related activities and tasks that would enable Nora to take increasing responsibility for herself as a thinking, moving human being, to enhance her understanding of her own ability to control herself within a given structure, and to aid her in moving beyond "do this for me" to "I can do it for myself".

In the early sessions major emphasis was placed on increasing Nora's range of locomotor and non-locomotor movement. A great deal of time was spent in developing effective two-way communication with Nora. Over the months our mutual progress was halting.

After four months of weekly sessions, on a "good" day, she was able to respond with appropriate movements when asked to do such things as swing her arms, shake her head, bend and stretch a leg, walk backwards, roll across a mat, or go turning around the room. While Nora does not consistently demonstrate her understanding of the following concepts, she has been exposed to all of them; loud, soft, begin (go), stop, same, different, shake, bend, stretch, move, less, apart, together, up, down, through, push, pull, long, short (duration), in, out, body parts, count, numbers (sequential and ordinal).

In many of the sessions Nora exhibited an exaggerated fear of me and/or the various movements she was asked to do. She often used such phrases as "You're going to hurt me; get away." Or, "Is this going to hurt me; I'm afraid." Nora would also step back from me, wrap her arms around her torso, and swing her body and head from side to side.

Even on good days Nora still showed less than full control over her movements, many of which were random. She appeared able to turn the movement on and off but lacked control to give continuity to the movement itself. The concept of tempo was chosen as a means to enable Nora to increasingly bring her movements under her own conscious control.

Nora was aware of the words fast, slow, and medium; yet it was difficult to assess what she understood them to mean. Sometimes I would ask her to move slowly and she would respond appropriately. In other sessions the request would be met with no response. The words fast and medium were also met with sporadic responses. We concluded that the tempo lesson plan should assume no reliable cognitive or kinesthetic understanding of these words.

LESSON PLAN	LESSON PRESENTATION
1. Two slow sounds on Orff (Nash 1974) xylophone. I do it, then Nora does it.	1. Nora, I'm going to make two sounds on the xylophone. Listen. Here's the mallet. No Nora, I'm not going to hurt you. Take the mallet. No, the mallet won't hurt you either. Good. Try making two sounds just like the ones you heard. OK. You keep that mallet. I have another one. Listen to the two sounds again. Nora, come on back down to the floor. No, you're all right. Come on back and try making those two sounds yourself.
2. Four fast sounds on xylophone. (Alternate Nora and me.)	2. Nora, listen to these sounds and then try making them yourself. OK, your turn. H-m-m. Listen and count how many sounds you hear this time. How many sounds were there? Right, four. Now you try it. Nora, I heard eight sounds that time. Listen to my sounds and then try it again. Count them out loud this time. No, Nora, I'm not going to hurt you. Listen to my four sounds. OK, your turn. Good. Do it again. Once more. Fine.
3. Two slow sounds. Compare with needle going into cloth when she's sewing	3. Let's go back to those two sounds again. Listen. Remember that piece of stitchery you showed me last week? I know you don't have it with you now, but, with just your hands can you show me how you move the needle. You're right. You don't have a needle. Pretend. Here, I have a pretend needle with me. You take it and show me how it moves in and out of the fabric. No this needle won't hurt you. Here, go ahead and try it. Yes, that's it. Push it in. Remember to pull it out on the other side. Good. Move the needle in and out a few more times. OK, I'll do it too. Yes, I have another needle. Nora, how are our needles moving. Right, they're moving in and out. How else are they moving? Yes, they're moving kind of slow. Here I'm going to play those two slow sounds on the xylophone again. No, I'm not going to hurt you. Have I hurt you before? OK then, you can still expect that I'm not going to hurt you. Nora, try pushing the needle in when you hear the first sound and pulling it out when you hear the second sound. Good, keep it going. Slow in, slow out . . ."
4. Four fast sounds. Compare to sewing machine needle going in and out of fabric.	4. Remember these four sounds? Sure, go ahead and play them. Hey, that's good. You have a sewing machine at your house don't you? Do you remember how the needle goes in and out of the fabric when you're using the machine? Is it like when you're sewing by hand? Yes, it is much faster. The needle moves fast just like the four sounds on the xylophone are fast. Try playing the four fast sounds again.

LESSON PLAN	LESSON PRESENTATION
5. Alternate two slow and four fast on xylophone.	5. Nora, let's try putting the slow and fast sounds together. First, there're two slow sounds, slow like hand-sewing. Second, there're four fast sounds like the machine sewing very fast. Let's both try making two slow and then four fast sounds. No Nora, It's OK for us to do it at the same time. Yes, I'm close to you. Am I hurting you? Come on, let's try it — two slow sounds, four fast sounds. One, two, ready, go . . . Let's make the slow sounds more slow. Good.
6. Add verbalization.	6. On the slow sounds let's say slow, and on the fast sounds let's say fast. OK, I'm a little tired too. Just try this and then we'll take a break. Here we go. Slow, slow. Fast, fast, fast, fast. Slow, slow. Fast, fast, fast, fast. Keep going by yourself. That's great! Let's take a break.
7. Two slow sounds using bend and stretch.	7. Nora, come on back to the floor. We're not sitting in chairs today. Of course you're going to be all right on the floor. You were OK when we were sitting on the floor before. Come on back. Remember when we were bending and stretching last week? What parts of your body did you bend and stretch? Yes, legs, neck, arms and, what's that called? It's the weird word that begins with a "t" sound. Right, torso. How about trying some bends and stretches with the xylophone sounds? Try the two slow sounds to begin with. At the first sound stretch your arm. When you hear the second sound, bend it. Take your time. It's like when you see instant replay on Monday night football, it's very slow. Slow stretch, slow bend. Ready? Stretch and bend, stretch and bend. Ready? Stretch and bend, stretch and bend. And stop. This time say the word "slow" with each stretch and bend. Listen for the xylophone. Go. Slow stretch, slow bend, slow stretch, slow bend. That's much better. Try the same thing with your other arm. Sure, go ahead and stand up. Fine. Can you slow stretch and slow bend both arms at the same time?"
8. Four fast sounds using bend and stretch.	8. I'd like for you to move with the four fast sounds now. Still bend and stretch, only this time it's fast. When you hear the first sound, stretch, second sound bend, third sound stretch, fourth sound bend. How many stretches is that? No, not four. Listen and watch while I do it. Listen for how many times I say stretch. Stretch, bend, stretch, bend. Right, two stretches. How many times did I say bend? Yes, there are two bends also. What body part do you want to move this time? Still arms? OK. Try it. Say stretch and bend while you do it. Listen for the xylophone. One, two, ready, go. That is fast. Try it again.
9. Combine one slow stretch-bend (two beats) with two fast stretch-bends (four beats).	9. Nora, here's the mallet again. Try playing two slow sounds and four fast sounds again. Sure, just keep on doing it as many times as you want. All right, I'll take over on the xylophone. Try the stretch and bend thing with both arms this time. That'll be slow stretch, slow bend, then what? Right, Stretch, bend, stretch, bend. That's how many fast movements? OK, we'll start with the slow stretch. Ready? And slow stretch, slow bend, then stretch, bend, stretch, bend. Again. Slow and slow, then fast, fast, fast, fast. Say it as you do it. Go.

LESSON PLAN

10. Slow—locomotor with xylophone.

11. Fast—locomotor with xylophone.

12. Slow-fast pattern—locomotor.

13. Introduce medium. Slow and fast on xylophone, then medium beat.

14. Fast, slow then medium with bend and stretch.

15. Define all as part of tempo.

16. All three tempi — locomotor with xylophone.

LESSON PRESENTATION

10. I'd like you to try some moving around the room now. How does that feel? Well, before you decide for sure that you don't want to do any more go over and see what I brought along for you to work with. Well it's OK to be afraid, but I don't think you'll find anything in the bag that'll frighten you. Go ahead and look. You can do it. What is it? Uh-huh, I thought you'd like a bigger scarf. The one last week was pretty small. Try moving with it however you want. Now hang onto the scarf but see if you can take just one step each time you hear a sound on the xylophone. Ready, and walk, walk, walk, walk, stay right with the sound. Walk, walk, walk, walk. OK. How are you moving? Yes, you're walking. Are you moving like a sewing machine? No, that's correct. You're walking slowly.

11. How about tying two corners of the scarf around your neck. That makes a great cape. You look super, especially with your shoulders back like that. Try moving with the music again, one step for each sound. Be careful, it might be different this time. Ready? And walk, walk, walk, walk, walk, walk, walk. And stop. How are you moving now? Right. Really fast. I liked the way you walked with the music even through it was so fast.

12. Remember this, two slow, four fast? Try walking with it. Ready and, slow, slow, fast, fast, fast, fast. You know what? You only moved fast. What happened to the slow walks at the beginning? Try it again. And, slow, slow. Stop. Let's just clap together. Two slow claps, four fast. And, clap slow . . . no Nora, the clapping won't hurt you. If it's too loud, let's clap softly, not too much noise. Ready and, slow and slow and fast, fast, fast, fast. All right, if the clapping scares you try just the walks. Listen for the xylophone. And, walk slow, walk slow, walk fast, fast, fast, fast. That's more like it, but you need to listen and stay right with the sound. Say slow and fast this time. Go. Good, that's better. Hey, I'm about finished, how about you?

During this session Nora was not in top form. She tended to drift in and out. Characteristically, she succeeded at some fairly complex tasks but had problems with others that seemed simple.

I did not get all the way through the lesson plan; working with an adult changes many of the ground rules for teaching. While we strive to design our teaching methods keeping the individuality and dignity of the learner in mind, the degree of autonomy that most adults perceive themselves to have requires more flexibility than does working with most children. I try to remember that Nora has the prerogative of walking out of the session. In earlier sessions Nora could manage to be near me only if both of us were seated in chairs. At first I felt that this might be because I am a man, but her reaction to Gertrude was often similar. One of our objectives in the most recent sessions was to gradually move away from the visible structure of chairs and tables without Nora's wanting to run out of the room. In this session she managed to stay in, but not without several close calls. At these junctures it was imperative that my investment in the lesson plan not exclude what was happening with Nora.

As she became obvious in this session, working with Nora is especially difficult when she becomes insecure and fearful. "You're going to hurt me" is Nora's way of dealing with Center clients and staff alike. The staff decided to minimize the impact of the behavior by directly answering no to her question, challenging her to look at another reality in the situation ("Have I hurt you before?"), or ignoring her question or comment entirely. By the time we reached step 7 in the lesson plan I was ignoring much of Nora's fear behavior. Sometimes it seemed to work. A short time later she and I were both beginning to feel fatigued, and I was desperately searching for alternatives. However, at the sound of the claps she became very agitated, covering her ears and screaming. I retreated quickly, jettisoning all three staff-determined responses and responding, instead, by trying to minimize the cause of her anxiety.

Seen in a larger perspective, Nora accomplished a great deal during this session. Her ability to focus and control her movement improved markedly. She was able to function more securely in a space without chairs or other large objects. She seemed to have mastered slow and fast in several different auditory, visual, vocal, cognitive, and kinesthetic ways. When we planned the next lesson, we decided to review this lesson and then expand and exchange the patterns Nora had mastered.

Through review we hope to determine if the learner retains accomplishments of the previous session. Variations on previous patterns reveal if the concepts can be generalized and the knowledge applied to a problem not previously encountered. When the learner demonstrates mastery of the concept in both situations, we are ready to move on to the next developmental sequence.

Developmental teaching of the whole person in a non-therapeutic mode leads the march for this Procession. The parade leader is supported by a process which contains assessment and analysis, the construction of a developmental sequence, and a detailed presentation and evaluation. Following in the line of march are examples of teaching *tempo* to a boy with cerebral palsy, a class of visually impaired boys and girls, and an adult who is mentally ill.

Learning is change through growth, and you must meet your students believing that you can produce growth through teaching. One can learn from experience, but as Vernon Law has said: "Experience is a hard teacher because she gives the test first, the lesson afterwards (Law 1960).

The Process reflects the adage: "The process is more important than the product; the journey is more significant than the destination." Many educators adhere ostensibly to this philosophy, but do not have the patience to withstand the slow, arduous trek. Thus they deny students the benefits of training.

To dance, the body must move from one design to another; to think, the mind must move from one idea to another. Trained bodies move with efficient coordination. Trained minds function rationally. With both trained mind and body, the student, handicapped or otherwise, has a movement foundation and problem-solving tools.

Some have bodies which can move or dance only in a limited way; some have minds which can move or think only in a limited way. In this Procession, body and mind can achieve their maximum movement and dance knowingly.

References

Blissymbolics Communication Foundation. *Blissymbolics.* Toronto, Canada: 862 Eglinton Avenue E., M4g 2L1. (No date.)

Boehm, Audrey. *Test of basic Concepts.* New York: Psychological Corporatioin, 1971.

Dolch, E. W. *Dolch Basic Sight Word Test.* Champagne, Illinois: Gerrard Publishing Co., 1942.

Law, Vernon. "How to be a Winner." *The National Sunday Magazine.* New York: United Newspapers Corporation, 1960.

Nash, Grace. *Creative Approaches to Child Development with Music, Language and Movement.* New York: Alfred Publishing Company, 1974.

12 Evolution of a Dance Program for Handicapped Children

Marcia L. Lloyd

My first contact with handicapped people and dance occurred when I was 12 and our dancing school took an Easter program to a residential home for the mentally retarded. Though we dancers worried about how we would be accepted, our fears were allayed when the audience clapped, whistled, and cheered after the first number. Some cried and we cried. We all accepted each other immediately. Memories of this experience have warmed me many times over throughout my life.

Later I researched dance activities for blind and deaf children as a final paper for a graduate course in adaptive physical education. During this project I discovered DANCE (Dance Activity Needed in a Child's Education) and corresponded with the founder. Learning about this organization formed in the eastern United States to give handicapped children a chance to dance, taught me that handicapped individuals need opportunities to dance for exercise, to express thought and feeling, and to enjoy moving just as nonhandicapped individuals do.

Still later the director of a child development center asked if I would try some of my dance activities with children enrolled in daily classes at the center. Was I interested? Yes. Could I do a good job? I thought so.

Questions flooded my mind. Would I be able to work with "those children?" With no previous experience, I wondered if the one special education course would get me started? Could I use the same approach with "special" children as with "normal" children? Would working with these children depress me? I knew some of the children would have no hope of living a normal life; others would be assimilated into public school classrooms, now referred to as mainstreaming.

Upon my first visit to the center I learned (1) chronological ages of children, (2) skill levels, (3) instructors' goals, (4) space and equipment available, (5) size of groups, and (6) staff expectations of a dance specialist.

Three groups with whom I could dance included a young group (ages 3-7 years), another group (ages 8-12 years), and the teenagers who eventually became my men dancers and included the man who was the aide.

I submitted a short pilot study to the director and the instructors, concerned that I might not have what it takes to succeed in this area. I quickly learned that I had the ability to care about people in the right way regardless of their handicaps. Believing that dance is at the heart of life, I had no choice but to share my belief with the students and staff at the center. I was hooked even before I had begun to dance with my new friends.

The Beginning

The proposal to work with the Child Development Center at Pocatello, Idaho was soon submitted and approved by the state. The pilot project designed for one class of 5-6 mobile children with chronological ages ranging from 2 years to 4 years began in 1973. A five-week session consisting of two lessons per week, 20-minutes per lesson was conducted. A short term project would allow me time to assess my feelings about working with the children and to evaluate the program. At the end of the five weeks written evaluations by the teacher and three aides who took part in the program were positive (I knew they would be) and recommendations to continue the program were emphatic.

The first five-week session was so successful that the program began to grow. When I discussed the dance program at a parents' meeting one evening, all of the parents wanted to see the program continued and gave me tremendous encouragement.

The Middle

By March 1973 two childrens' groups were taking part in the dance program twice a week, with the second group of older children who were able to do more activities. By June each group could perform at least five activities. Some circle games — "Ring Around the Rosy," "Looby Loo," and "Did You Ever See a Lassie" — were favorites. But when all else failed, we used scarves to create our own choreographies to a series of musical selections. The scarves seemed to make the children feel more secure, and they concentrated on trying to make the scarf move high and low, fast and slow, in circles and any other ways they could imagine. There was always one of us with a scarf over our head "hiding."

Everyone loved to beat the drum or gong. The gong was a large lid from a flour container suspended from a string in a hole near the top. The gong has continued to give an excellent sound. The cost was minimal as the flour bin and lid were given to me by a bakery owner.

In June 1973, I held an in-service training session for aides and teachers who would be working with the children through the summer months while I was away. Returning to the Center in September, I was delighted to learn the dance activities had continued and some teachers had gained enough confidence to try their own rhythmic movement ideas. Another class was requested. Now three classes received dance activities twice weekly. In January 1974 we added a fourth class.

In March 1974, we began a 30 minute weekly dance class for teenagers with chronological ages from 13-17 years. The nine dance sessions ran from 20-30 minutes per group depending on the attention span of the group on a given day. The younger children seemed to be able to participate for 20 minutes, and I spent 30 minutes with the teenage group of eleven boys and three girls.

The Program

The program was based primarily on large muscle movements because the students spent most of their time sitting with therapists individually or with their group to develop speech, hearing, and manual dexterity. I endeavored to help each child become more aware of body parts (head, shoulders, arms, hands, chest, stomach, legs, feet, toes, and fingers), the body in space, the relationship to other bodies in space. Because the children's attendance at the Center varied, each session was complete. I also built on each lesson so children could become secure with the familiar, then gradually added new activities and skills. As children developed favorite activities, requests were welcomed and encouraged.

Stretching and bending, locating body parts, locomotor movements to music or percussive instruments, using scarves to help create large movements, and bean bags on heads for balance are a few of the skills used in the dance program. Halloween, Thanksgiving, Christmas, Valentine's Day, and Easter provided movement themes.

The values of the program grew with increased contact with students and teachers. The attention span of the participants increased. Following the third session with the teenagers, the teacher reported that they were working better as a group than ever before. Teachers and aides benefitted from the program as well, stating they felt better and more energetic yet relaxed after dance sessions. The teachers noted that the children seemed more relaxed, attentive, and more cooperative.

My notes on the "happenings" after each session include:
"R. wandered a lot, but smiled and tried arm circles and clapping knees and hands . . . C. tried very hard, but seemed to enjoy activities, could roll. (I was sad to learn that cystic fibrosis took C. from us.) . . . MJ. came out from under the table today and joined us in one activity. . .

D. let me hold his hand today for the first time." By keeping a log of important activities, I became aware of progress when I reread my notes.

Never was I depressed while working with these children because, immersed in watching for the slightest progress and memory development, I was never disappointed in their performances. The entire program was an ego trip for me.

I also kept brief notes on music and activities and evaluated each session. As I reread my notebooks, I found: "Children really seemed to respond well and enjoy the music today . . . seems that activities are limited due to physical problems or age of children. . . . I need to add a new activity next time." Most rewarding in the three year project was a note made on the seventh lesson of the first year: "All of the children are extremely responsive. Each one tries so hard and lets me work with them individually. Some of the children give me a kiss and a hug hello and goodbye."

Children in the Program

The children in the program had various disabilities or handicaps including the usual pattern of multi-handicaps. Some had cystic fibrosis, hearing loss, sight problems, or birth defects such as cerebral palsy, and all had speech problems. Various degrees of mental retardation were found in all children who came to the center.

The teachers and I agreed that no child would be forced to participate in the dance sessions. Instead we attempted to have so much fun that children would choose to join. As the dance program developed, nonparticipators usually chose to join in the following steps: (1) child refuses to participate (2) shares in one activity then leaves (3) begins to share in more activities as attention span increases, and (4) participates almost completely in the dance lesson. The goal of the dance program was movement for all who could and would participate.

The following comments recorded in my notebook reveal the progress of some children in the program.

D. about age 10. "Did not allow anyone to hold his hand during the first few sessions. Gradually he felt more comfortable with the dance teacher—began to respond by allowing physical contact. He seemed to enjoy the activities more and spent more time with the group. Still has a problem with coordination—sight problems—cannot be assimilated into a public school setting."

M. age 12. "Spent the first few sessions screaming a high pitched scream. As the program progressed she quieted down; less and less screaming occurred until finally she participated in a complete session without inappropriate sounds. She became a most enjoyable student and helped reinforce in the dance teacher's mind that the children can remember various dances. M. also reached the point of selecting favorite activities and requesting these each time we met. She increased her coordination markedly. Her socialization skills rose dramatically."

MJ age 4. "Participated in the pilot program. During the first few lessons she stayed under the table (her observation room). Success was getting her out from under the table. Eventually she came out and began spending a few moments with the group, but allowed no physical contact, not even hand holding. After a year of dance activity she had made great strides — emerged from under the table, allowed some hand holding, began to verbalize once in a while. After two years, MJ moved to an older class and has increased her attention span for dance as well as other activities. She allows the dance teacher and other children to hold her hand most of the time. She exhibits her joy and excitement for her favorite dance activities either by verbalization or jumping up and down (like any of the rest of us)! She appointed herself collector of the bean bags following one of the activities. (A further note on MJ, by 1979 she had been mainstreamed into a local elementary classroom of special education children).

K. age 12. "Spent a year in the dance program. He spent his first several sessions running around the room and screaming, refusing to join the dance group. The dance teacher doubted if he would choose to take part—surprise—he joined the group after six weeks and shared one activity. Then he began spending more and more time with the group until he reached about 90 percent participation."

S. age 8. "After being part of the class for a month, he decided to spend less time running around in small circles. He began to observe the activities of the other children and imitated acceptable behavior. He seems to be enjoying the dance activities and is learning that he can move slowly as well as fast. He's gaining control of his body and can stop and start without falling down. He has no apparent physical disabilities.

A Fond Farewell—but a Sad Goodbye

I was employed by the state on an hourly basis for ten hours per week; the wages were suitable. The first two years went well and I annually reported the progress of the program. During the third year, I was asked to write three reports to explain the program benefits and progress, and to justify its existence. I was always happy to write these reports because the benefits and progress of all who were involved was obvious. But when I completed the third report, I knew the program and my job were in jeopardy. News of program cutting—especially of programs considered to be "frills"—came daily. Then in May 1975 I learned the dance program had been cut. With Title IX and Public Law 94-142, the student body changed and many programs were cut or rearranged; students were mainstreamed.

One of the joys of my dance activities with handicapped children at the center has been seeing many of these children taking part in regular public school classroom activities. As they run across the playground I somehow feel they are better prepared because of the dance they had earlier in their lives.

My only regret was the attitude taken by those in charge of program cutting. The belief that dance programs are "frills" and can be done away with is not a local problem; it must be dealt with on a larger scale. Individually, however, we must each be a persuasive force to show that dance is the heart of life, and every life, especially of the handicapped, should have the opportunity to dance.

The Future

Despite program cuts, many opportunities will continue because dance is increasing for all ages and abilities. Increased awareness of the use of dance for the handicapped is apparent by the number of books and articles that are being published. More workshops train personnel in dance for the handicapped. More teachers than ever before are using dance with handicapped individuals. Fun, exercise, the personal satisfaction of self-expression, and the rewarding use of leisure time all favor dance for persons with handicapping conditions.

References

Cratty, Bryant. *Movement, Perception and Thought*. Palo Alto, CA: Peek Publications, 1970.

Hackett, Layne. *Movement Exploration and Games for the Mentally Retarded*. Peek Publications.

Hackett, Layne and Robert Jenson. *A Guide to Movement Exploration*. Peek Publications.

Robins, Ferris and Jenet. *Educational Rhythmics for Mentally and Physically Handicapped Children*. New York: Association Press, 1968.

13 Simplified Movement Behavior Analysis As a Basis for Designing Dance Activities for the Handicapped

Sally Fitt

This chapter illustrates how simple analysis of individuals' use of time, space, and force can function in planning movement and dance activities for the handicapped. The word simplified in the title is used because "full blown" movement behavior analysis requires considerable preparation and study, yet teachers of the handicapped may easily apply basic concepts and principles.

For purposes of clarification, handicapped is used here to indicate individuals who have some form of physical, mental, or emotional limitation. Everyone has limitations; the only difference between individuals who are labeled "normal" and those labelled "handicapped" is the severity and/or the visibility of the limitation. Even though I have some reservations about labeling individuals handicapped (since some handicapped are less limited than normals), the word handicapped is used in this article for ease of communication.

Breakdown of Skills Necessary for Teaching Handicapped

Any teaching requires the ability to analyze the skills to be taught and to identify their basic elements. Moreover, if the teacher does not identify and begin teaching at the skill level of students, it is unlikely that learning will follow. For teachers of the handicapped, accurately assessing students' skill level is even more critical than for nonhandicapped, because learning skills must be reduced to very small steps in order to insure the students' success. It is necessary to tell teachers of the handicapped how important successful experiences are to their students. For some handicapped individuals, success is relatively new; yet we all know that success is possible if the expectations are reasonable and possible. Dance skills frequently thought of as basic in "normal" classes — such as plies, jumps, leaps, walks, runs, or hops—are actually high level complicated skills. The customary system for breaking down skills into their simplest form is not nearly basic enough. One must look at movement skills from a different perspective.

Basic Elements of Movement

The basic elements of motion are *time, space,* and *force.* (Hunt 1964; Laban and Lawrence 1947). Although full analysis of an individual's characteristic use of time, space and force can become a highly specialized skill (Dell 1970; Fitt and Hanson 1978), it is possible to effectively use an abbreviated analysis to identify basic movement needs of the handicapped. By focusing on the particular combination of time, space, and force used in a given skill, the teacher can isolate critical components necessary to perform that skill. In a jump for example, the extension of the knee, hip, and ankle must be strong (force) and fast (time); to be effective, the space must be relatively small or the jump will go off in all directions simultaneously. A student who cannot quickly activate the muscles of the knee, hip, and ankle will have little chance of jumping well. Even this brief example suggests lead-up activities to prepare the student to jump. If the teacher has carefully analyzed the target skills, systematically observed a student's characteristic movement patterns, and then designed learnings to prepare for performing the skill, success is more probable than through a shotgun approach to dance teaching. Critical in this process is a clear understanding of the kinesiological functioning of the human body. The intent of this chapter, however, is to discuss basic movement behavior analysis so as to facilitate more effective learning for handicapped students.

Movement Behavior: Definition and Purpose

Movement behavior is the analysis and identification of qualitative movement patterns characteristic of an individual or group. The focus is on the *style* of performance rather than the skill or the effectiveness. By observing an individual's use of time, space, and force in many different situations, the movement behavior specialist can consolidate these observations into a movement behavior profile which illustrates the individual's characteristic pattern (central tendency), the breadth of that pattern (range), and finally the characteristic capacities and limitations. Four basic assumptions are involved in movement behavior analysis:

1) The human being operates as a functional whole: mind, emotions, and body are not separate from each other.
2) Each individual has a characteristic and unique pattern of movement behavior.
3) Movement behavior patterns reflect other behavior patterns of the individual including personality.
4) It is possible to expand the range of an individual's movement behavior.

The core of a movement behavior program lies in these four assumptions; its central objective is *to facilitate the participant's development of the fullest possible range of movement patterns.* Movement behavior programs therefore seek to expand movement potential after identifying basic limitations through systematic observation[1] (Fitt and Hanson 1978; Buchannan 1970; Hanson 1970; Fitt 1974).

A Conceptual Model of Movement Behavior

The theoretical model of movement behavior (Hunt 1964; Fitt and Hanson 1978; Fitt 1975) includes much more than the analysis of an individual's use of time, space, and force which is the focus of this chapter. To give the reader a sense of the scope of

---

[1]The film, A Time to Move, documents the growth shown by a group of "normal" children who participated in the Movement Behavior Program at University Elementary School, UCLA, Los Angeles. The film is available for purchase or rental from: Special Purpose Films, 26740 Latigo Shore Dr., Malibu, CA 90265.

Figure 1 Theoretical Model of Movement Behavior

I. The Analysis of Movement Behavior
  A. Quantitative Analysis

The focus of this chapter.
  1. Time: Slow . . . . . Fast
  2. Space: Personal: Small . . . . Large
        Environmental: Small . . . . Large
  3. Force: Weak . . . . Strong

  B. Qualitative Analysis
  1. Time: Rhythm: Regular . . . . Irregular
        Pace: Accelerating . . . Steady . . . Decelerating
  2. Space: Path: Straight . . . . Curved
        Shape: Straight . . . . Curved
        Direction: Forward, Backward, Sideward, Across the Midline,
              Upward, Downward, Inward, Outward
  3. Force: Focus: Intense . . . .Diffuse
        Weight Management: Resistant . . . Indulgent
  4. Neuromuscular Excitation Patterns (Hunt 1970; Fitt 1975)

II. The Analysis of Perceptual Modes
  A. Body Image
  B. Figure-Ground Perception (Field Dependent and Field Independent)
  C. Spatial Perception
  1. Laterality
  2. Perception of the Horizontal
  3. Perception of the Vertical
  D. Brain hemispheric dominance

III. The Analysis of Expressive Modes
  A. Gestures
  B. Postures
  C. Facial Expression
  D. Graphics
  E. Residual Neuromuscular Tension Patterns (Rathbone 1943)

IV. The Relationship between Movement Behavior and Perceptual Modes

V. The Relationship between Movement Behavior and Expressive Modes

VI. The Relationship between Perceptual Modes and Expressive Modes

Figure 2. The Interrelationship of the Elements of the Conceptual Model in the Movement Behavior Profile

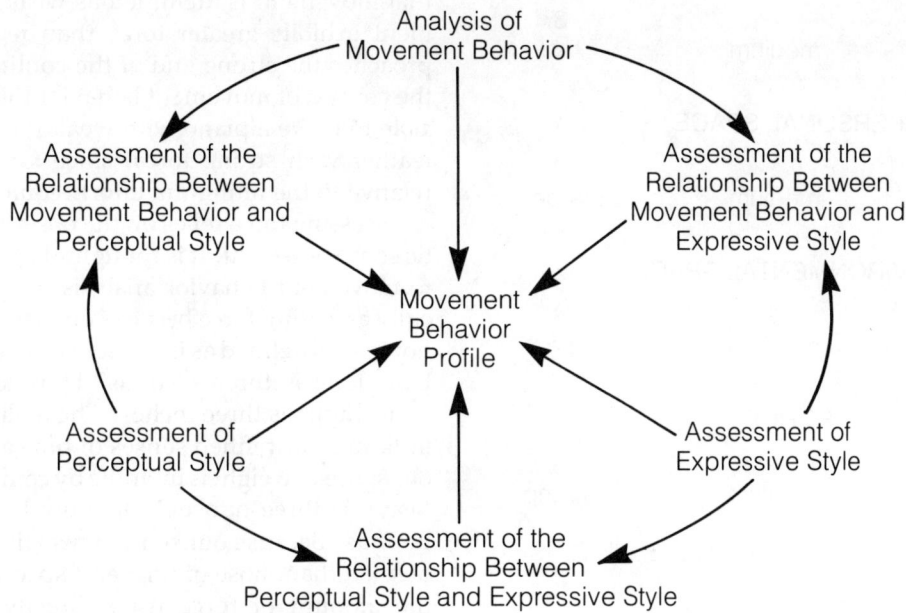

```
                        Analysis of
                     Movement Behavior

  Assessment of the                          Assessment of the
  Relationship Between                       Relationship Between
  Movement Behavior and                      Movement Behavior and
  Perceptual Style                           Expressive Style

                        Movement
                        Behavior
                        Profile

  Assessment of                              Assessment of
  Perceptual Style                           Expressive Style

                   Assessment of the
                  Relationship Between
           Perceptual Style and Expressive Style
```

movement behavior, the full model (to date, for somehow it continues to grow) is illustrated in Figures 1 and 2. Only Section IA of the model is used in the simplified analysis.

After studying Figures 1 and 2, the reader will realize that this chapter focuses on a small portion of comprehensive movement behavior analysis. Yet even the simplified form can yield much information to the teacher of dance for the handicapped.

The Process of Observation

Observation of movement behavior elements, like any systematic form of observation, requires practice. Dance teachers constantly observe movement behavior, but their observations may be unsystematic and intuitive. Systematic observation requires labeling, defining, and recording variables observed. Based on elements from the movement behavior model, the simplified observation focuses on:

Time

slow . . . . .fast

Space

small . . . . .large

Force

weak . . . . .strong

Each of these elements is quantitative: the amount of time used or performance duration, the amount of space used or movement size, and the amount of force used in the management of weight

The Initial Stages of Observation

When initiating movement behavior observation, it is frequently necessary to focus on only one element at a time. The observer might best begin by looking at the time component of movement because our highly developed sense of time in this culture makes us aware of subtle variances in use of time. Simplifying further, the observer should first classify movements according to a three point scale: slow, medium, or fast (see Figure 3). This can be expanded to a seven point scale as observation skills become more refined.

A critical factor in movement behavior analysis is that assessment of time, (and space and force as well) is *relative*. How fast is fast? How slow is slow? The reference point upon which judgment is based is *human potential for the task being observed*. How fast can a human being possibly walk? How slowly? The referent for a walk obviously will be different than for a run. One assesses each movement relative to the human potential for that skill. With experience

Figure 3. The Three Point Observation Scale

TIME

| 1 | 2 | 3 |
| slow | medium | fast |

PERSONAL SPACE

| 1 | 2 | 3 |
| small | medium | large |

ENVIRONMENTAL SPACE

| 1 | 2 | 3 |
| small | medium | large |

FORCE

| 1 | 2 | 3 |
| weak | medium | strong |

the reference points become more refined. Movements initially classified as fast may appear less so when one observes even faster movements. Here one naturally moves to the more refined seven point rating system which offers more precise distinctions.

An observer who can assess movement speed may proceed to the next variable, space. Space must be divided into personal and environmental space. Personal space is the space immediately surrounding the mover through which he or she can move without using locomotor movements such as walking, running, crawling. Environmental space is the space used which requires locomotion. Because a person might use small personal space and large environmental space or vice versa, it is necessary to assess a mover's use of both personal and environmental space. The assessment of use of space, like time, requires a task-specific reference point. The amount of personal and environmental space used in writing a letter is different from that used in sweeping a floor. Again, as the observer develops increasingly refined observations the use of the seven point scale will follow naturally.

The final variable is force. Possibly the most difficult variable for the first time observer, the force of a movement is not directly related to the strength of the mover. Assessing force requires two observations in movement behavior: the minimum force

necessary to do the movement and the actual force used. Force is assessed *relative to the minimum amount of force required to perform the task*. If a mover uses minimum force to perform a movement task, that movement is identified as weak. If the movement exhibits greater force than required, it approaches the strong end of the continuum. Within the context of movement behavior theory, it is possible to move a piano with weak force and to lift a feather with strong force, since force is assessed relative to the minimum effort required.

Assessing force relies on the observer's kinesthetic sense of weight. It is thought that the newcomer to movement behavior analysis has greatest difficulty assessing force because our sense of weight is not as well defined as is our sense of time and space. How long is three seconds? How far away from your thumb is three inches? The ability to estimate indicates our refined senses of time and space. Yet our sense of weight is infantile by comparison. How heavy is three ounces? Or, how heavy is twelve pounds? Because our sense of weight is less clearly defined than those of time and space, and because the amount of force used directly depends on weight, assessing force is, at first, more difficult.

Because it is difficult to guide new observers without demonstrating specific movements, they must *begin observing*. First observations will require revising what one records as fast or slow, large and small, and weak and strong. With experience, however, one will develop a sense of the potential range for different movements.

A Common Problem in Observation

As the observer develops reference points for assessing relative speed, size and force of movement, the tendency is to make one's own movement patterns or experience the reference point, rather than relying on knowledge of human movement potential. Yet our own movement patterns may not include a full range of elements. If the observer consistently uses slow time, for example, many movements which appear fast may be closer to medium speed. Realizing how personal movement behavior patterns affect accurate observations requires an observer to guard against letting those experiential biases distort objective observation. By observing as many people in different situations as possible, one develops a sense of the possible range for each variable and clarifies referents for each variable. Practice observations with more than one observer are helpful. Common observation is then sharpened through use of the seven point scale, illustrated in Figure 4.

Figure 4. The Seven Point Scale (Hunt 1964)

TIME

1	2	3	4	5	6	7
slow			medium			fast

PERSONAL SPACE

1	2	3	4	5	6	7
small			medium			large

ENVIRONMENTAL SPACE

1	2	3	4	5	6	7
small			medium			large

FORCE

1	2	3	4	5	6	7
weak			medium			strong

The Second Phase of Observation

The second phase of observation involves intensive observation of a single individual. The observer selects a subject who can easily be observed in many different situations. Using the seven point scale (Figure 4) the observer identifies the amount of time, space, and force used by recording hatch marks (卅) directly below the number which corresponds to the amount used. As the observer views more of the subject's movements, the simplified movement behavior profile takes shape; consistencies appear. New observers often ask "How much observation is enough?" When a pattern becomes apparent, new observations substantiate that pattern, and further observation reveals no new information, the observer usually can begin the profile. (I hesitate. New information is always possible, but one *must* stop somewhere.)

The Simplified Movement Behavior Profile

The movement behavior profile records all observations, consolidating records onto a single profile sheet for assessment. If the observer has used the same form for each observation, the profile is automatically completed when the observations cease. Otherwise it is necessary to compile observations on a single form. Two different movement behavior profiles, included in Figures 5 and 6, illustrate two individuals' capacities and limitations.

Analysis of the Profiles

Using the two profiles, above, one can easily identify gaps in each person's movement behavior. Although these two profiles may seem to illustrate extreme differences, each profiles a "normal" child whom I observed and worked with at University Elementary School at UCLA. I have changed the names.

Ruth was a little girl who seemed to be encased in a fog. Her consistent use of weak force slow time contributed to and reinforced this condition. Her use of space was interesting, for she used small to medium personal space, but medium to large environmental space. Her movements never extended to the full range of her personal space; her arms flopped and floated (weak and slow) fairly close to her torso. Similarly her legs moved loosely (weak) and lackadaisically (slow) while never moving out to their full range in space (small). Her use of environmental space was quite large, however, as she meandered over the playground or classroom, leaving personal belongings for teachers and aids to pick up and return to her locker.

Dennis, like a stick of dynamite looking for a place to explode, was a different story entirely. While not officially labeled "hyperactive," his movement behavior patterns could be so interpreted. Dennis seldom walked either in the classroom or playground. He ran, jumped, hopped, using characteristically fast, strong, and large movements.

Figure 5. Simplified Movement Behavior Profile — Ruth

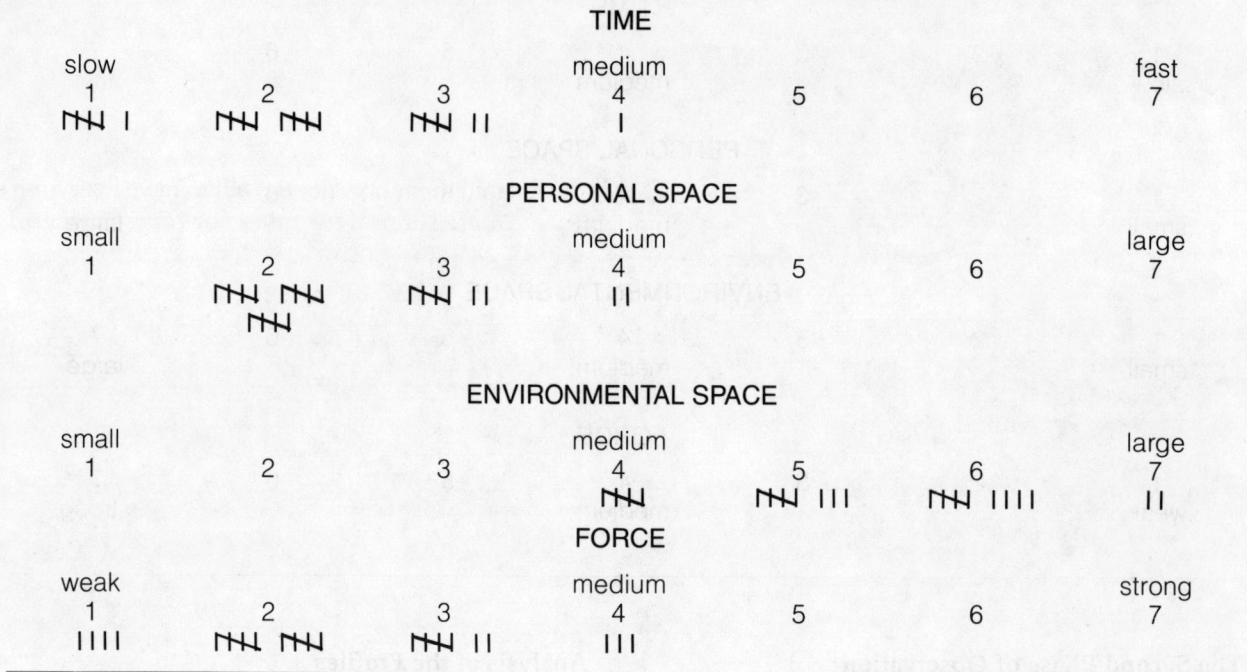

TIME

slow			medium			fast
1	2	3	4	5	6	7
ᚷᚷᚷ I	ᚷᚷᚷ ᚷᚷᚷ	ᚷᚷᚷ II	I			

PERSONAL SPACE

small			medium			large
1	2	3	4	5	6	7
	ᚷᚷᚷ ᚷᚷᚷ ᚷᚷᚷ	ᚷᚷᚷ II	II			

ENVIRONMENTAL SPACE

small			medium			large
1	2	3	4	5	6	7
			ᚷᚷᚷ	ᚷᚷᚷ III	ᚷᚷᚷ IIII	II

FORCE

weak			medium			strong
1	2	3	4	5	6	7
IIII	ᚷᚷᚷ ᚷᚷᚷ	ᚷᚷᚷ II	III			

Figure 6. Simplified Movement Behavior Profile — Dennis

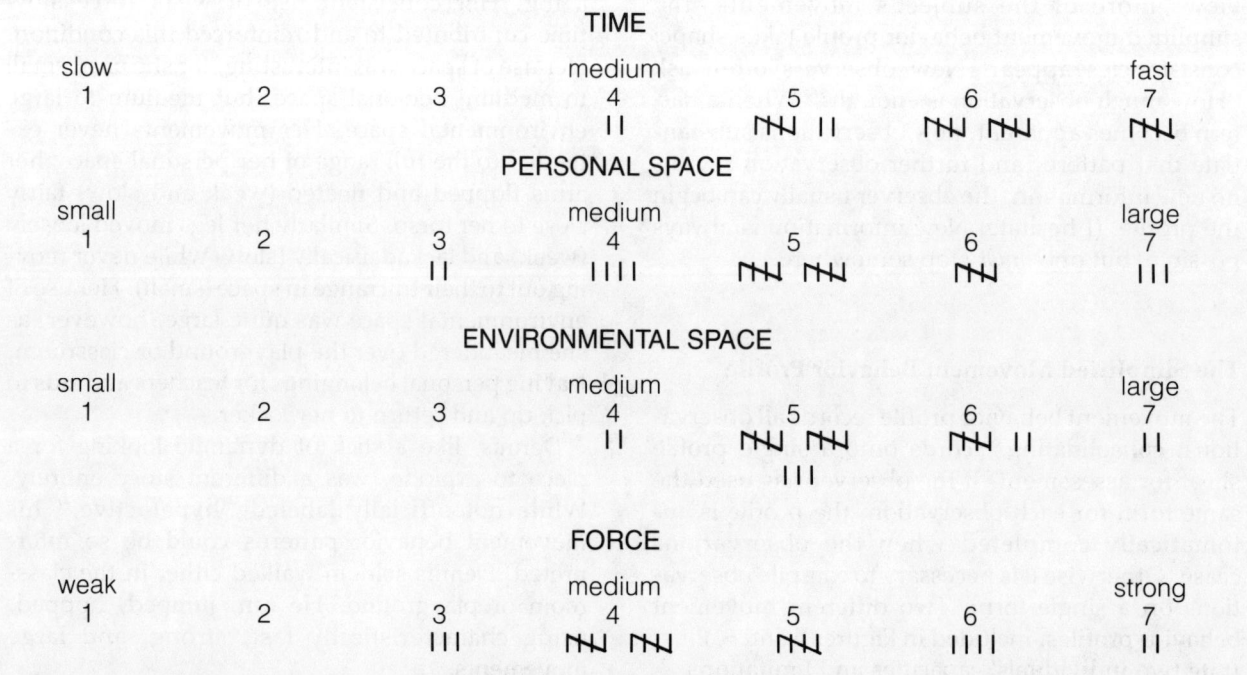

TIME

slow			medium			fast
1	2	3	4	5	6	7
			II	ᚷᚷᚷ II	ᚷᚷᚷ ᚷᚷᚷ	ᚷᚷᚷ

PERSONAL SPACE

small			medium			large
1	2	3	4	5	6	7
		II	IIII	ᚷᚷᚷ ᚷᚷᚷ	ᚷᚷᚷ	III

ENVIRONMENTAL SPACE

small			medium			large
1	2	3	4	5	6	7
			II	ᚷᚷᚷ ᚷᚷᚷ	ᚷᚷᚷ II	II
			III			

FORCE

weak			medium			strong
1	2	3	4	5	6	7
		III	ᚷᚷᚷ ᚷᚷᚷ	ᚷᚷᚷ	IIII	II

Although both children were intellectually capable, neither was able to work effectively at a task for any extended time. Ruth drifted into a task briefly and then wandered off before she had time to learn anything. Dennis, on the other hand, could not slow down long enough to process any information. He stopped briefly at a table, only to jump up quickly and be off to something else.

Designing Movement Experiences from the Profiles

The movement experiences designed for these two children were very different. Ruth's movement assignments, designed to increase her ability to focus on a task without "spacing out," included an obstacle course with a tunnel made from classroom chairs and a cardboard tube about two feet in diameter. Encouraged and enticed to crawl through the tunnel, she had to use stronger force than usual to get through it, and the obstacle course provided an external focus for her.

We also used the obstacle course for Dennis, with a different movement objective. Instructed not to "pop" out of the chair tunnel halfway through, he was forced to slow down, since there was no way to navigate the obstacle course rapidly.

These specifically designed objectives expanded Dennis' and Ruth's movement behavior patterns. The techniques of observation, assessment, and design of objectives can be equally effective with the handicapped, for the variables of motion observed are the most basic elements of movement.

Special Uses of Movement Behavior Analysis for the Handicapped

In addition to work with individuals, it is also possible to identify group movement characteristics. Pertinent questions to be answered by systematic observation follow:

Are there movement behavior patterns that are characteristic of the deaf or hearing impaired?

Are there patterns that are characteristic of the blind?

Are there patterns that are characteristic of the cerebral palsied individual?

Are there patterns that are characteristic of arthritics?

Can movement experiences be more effectively designed when one is aware of the characteristic patterns of these groups?

What movement experiences will offer opportunities for success for each individual in a group?

These questions are included to encourage the reader to probe possible applications of simplified movement behavior analysis. While many research projects could be designed around the use of simplified movement behavior, the potential of movement analysis will go unused unless teachers of the handicapped begin to observe relative time, space, and force used in their students' movement. That will not happen by osmosis. The teacher must make a conscious effort to develop skills necessary for effective observation. That can only happen if *you* begin observing *now*.

References

Buchannan, Edith, "The Relationship of Affective Behavior to Movement Patterns, Body Image, and Visual Perception in Four and Five-Year-Old Children." Los Angeles: Unpublished Doctoral Dissertation, UCLA, 1970.

Dell, Cecily, *A Primer for Movement Description*. New York: Dance Notation Bureau, 1970.

Fitt, Sally S., "The Assessment of Inter-rater Agreement and Validity of Observation Techniques for the Identification of Neuromuscular Excitation Patterns." Los Angeles: Unpublished Doctoral Dissertation, UCLA, 1975.

Fitt, Sally S., "The Individual and His Environment." *School Review*. Volume 82, Number 4, pp. 617-620, 1974.

Fitt, Sally S. and Hanson, Deanna S., *Movement Behavior Programs for Young Children*. Fitt Distributing, 2486 Nantucket Drive, Salt Lake City, Utah 84121, 1978.

Fitt, Sally S., "The Use of Simplified Movement Behavior Analysis As A Basis for Inferring Internal Events." Unpublished Paper, 1974.

Hanson, Deanna S., "The Effect of A Concentrated Program in Movement Behavior on the Affective Behavior of Four-Year-Old Children At University Elementary School." Los Angeles: Unpublished Doctoral Dissertation, UCLA, 1970.

Hunt, Valerie V., "Movement Behavior: A Model for Action." *Quest*. Monograph II. Spring, 1964. pp. 69-91.

Hunt, Valerie, V., "The Neuromuscular Structuring of Human Energy." Araminta Little, ed. *Proceedings of the Forty-Fifth Conference of the Western Society for Physical Education of College Women*, 1970.

Laban and Lawrence, *Effort*. London: Macdonald and Evans Co., 1947.

Rathbone, Josephine, *Relaxation*. New York: Teacher's College, Columbia University, 1943.

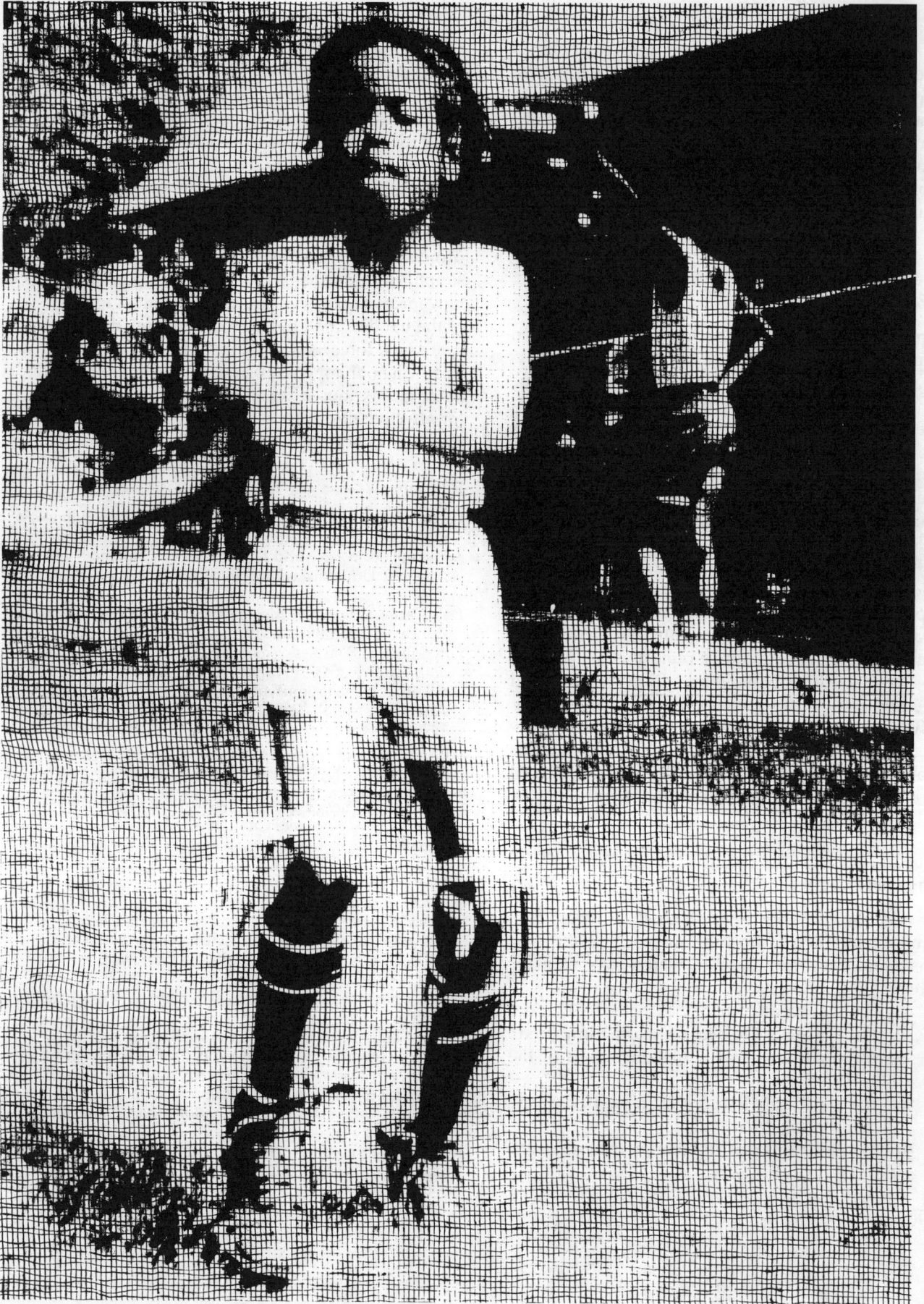

14 Dance for the Handicapped Child: Pitfalls or Conquests?

Faith Clark

There are many who feel they were born before their time. Twenty-five years ago I would have especially welcomed a monograph devoted to dance for the handicapped. At that time, I had the privilege of meeting the great pioneer of dance therapy, Marian Chace. The more I learned about her work with psychiatric patients at St. Elizabeth's Hospital in Washington, D.C., the more intrigued I became with the idea of using dance as therapy for those with physical disabilities. The idea remained dormant until I read *Karen* by Marie Killilea (1952). The book tells of Karen's parents' desperate search for alternatives to institutionalizing their cerebral palsied child. I was impressed with "Dr. B's" therapeutic program for Karen, and determined to sleuth out the doctor's real name. When I located Dr. Phelps, we discussed my dreams about dance and therapy, and I was invited to work with him and his staff as a learner.

Although Dr. Phelps may not have felt I was qualified to work with the handicapped, he wisely let me learn this for myself. Assigned as an aide to the head therapist, I was invited to attend staff planning sessions and was given material on C.P. to study. Later, I worked with two children directly. The first child, a beautiful but severely retarded ataxic, could walk only between parallel bars; her ataxia was so severe she could not release her hands to turn to walk the other way. The therapist and I devised a sand-bagged baby carriage so she could travel about the center's grounds with greater freedom, and I was assigned to go with her. This represented great progress for the patient who enjoyed the movement, but this was not the dance therapy I had hoped to do.

The second child was a young teenager with severe spasticity who dreamed of learning ballet. I tried to adapt the classical form to her movement patterns but quickly became frustrated. With great timing and intuition, Dr. Phelps sent me to a nearby public school with an excellent therapy program for the physically handicapped where I observed two other children. The therapist there explained how eager but unknowing dance teachers had compounded each child's handicap. The message was clear: don't try to help with problems you don't understand. To alleviate my discouragement Dr. Phelps outlined the steps that would allow me to pursue my goals, suggesting I return to school to study therapy and then ally myself with a specialist, hospital, or school dedicated to work with the handicapped. Since I did not have the funds to pursue further schooling, I devoted myself to my other great love, creative movement for children.

Some years later, conducting a three week teachers' workshop in creative movement in Billings, Montana, the special education teacher asked me to work with her brain damaged children. She asked me to relate the experiences to their special study of insects. Realizing I could not further complicate their handicaps physically, I tried. The six to eight children responded enthusiastically to the activities. But as I was ignorant of the great variations in behavior caused by brain damage, in less time than it takes to tell this story, each child was off on a totally unrelated activity. When I enlisted my workshop group to work with me to permit one-to-one encounters, learning began to take place. This class became the project of the workshop, from which we all learned. Confession is great for the soul, but the main purpose here is to emphasize the need for dance for the handicapped and the equal need for special knowledge, methods, and materials. Although I never returned to school for training, I have followed and supported the dance therapy movement.

Only 38 years ago in 1942, Marion Chace began her work. The American Dance Therapy Association, 13 years old, established a registry and standards for dance therapists eight years ago. Dance therapy pioneers gave long years of experimental work under the guidance of gifted doctors and therapists.

The Purpose of Dance For The Handicapped

I would ask those who wish to teach dance to the handicapped to examine their purpose. Is the dance to be recreational, an addition to the physical education program, or a creative arts experience? Is the teacher trying to expose children to a specific dance form or to help them adjust to living? The great danger is in attempting too much through the dance experience and accomplishing too little.

Claire Schmais discusses the difference between teaching dance to the handicapped and dance therapy in a JOHPER article (Schmais 1976). She cities a historic confusion owing to dance therapy pioneers being dance teachers before they became dance therapists. Shifting from their studios or classrooms to work in clinics and hospitals, they developed the special skills which came to define the new profession of dance therapy. Yet if the principal intent is to teach a specific dance form, however therapeutic the results, one practices dance teaching. The dance therapist, in contrast, uses dance to establish a relationship that will evolve toward therapeutic ends.

Today many dance programs for the handicapped are connected with hospitals, clinics, special schools, rehabilitation centers, sheltered workshops, mental health programs, public schools, and in dance studios. In most programs the dance teacher can get advice and guidance from doctors and therapists. Persons attempting to build programs in the public schools or in their studios without special background for this work should beware for they can be sued for malpractice.

Children with handicapping conditions do not need further setbacks. Before working with any handicapped child the teacher should know the answers to the following questions: What is the prognosis for the particular handicap? How can the child be helped? What might adversely affect the child? How do structural and functional disabilities differ and what is the proper way to deal with each? Which handicaps, or their stages, require one to one teaching? At what point may children be taught in groups? Which children are ready for mainstreaming? What is the proper length of a class for each teaching method? Which dance forms are best for specific handicaps? Are structured experiences or problem solving approaches more beneficial?

Background Needed for Dance for the Handicapped

Certain foundational knowledge is important in working with all students, such as anatomy, kinesiology, child growth and development, psychology, and motor learning. Body mechanics, physiology, and human behavior would further aid the prospective teacher of dance for the handicapped. Those interested in working with dance for the handicapped must avail themselves of a variety of forms including modern, folk, jazz, social, ethnic, ballet, and creative dance for children. The handicapped child needs excellence in skills less than the basic fulfillment found in moving.

Following study, the prospective teacher should teach "normal" children a year or more to develop skill and confidence in dance teaching, to observe movement problems encountered by all learners, and to develop skill in adapting movement to an individual's body type, balance, and alignment. Study of Rudolph Laban's effort-shape theory has helped many dance teachers work with movement more effectively.

While some handicaps seem easier to work with than others, each requires methods and materials specific to that handicapping condition. An example is teaching deaf students. Peter Wisher states communication is one of the greatest problems for the teacher of the deaf, (Wisher 1974), and the teacher must learn one of the five methods commonly practiced. Wisher, however, feels that the simultaneous method which combines lip reading, fingerspelling, signing, and speech reading is most effective. Adaptions will need to be made in teaching methods, but not in the physical skills of dance. Traditional accompaniment may be adapted or dispensed with when it is not important to the dance ideas. Smaller rooms, enclosed spaces, and wooden floors help increase the vibrations of percussive sound cues. Other methods of teaching and the forms of dance are the same as for the hearing child. Creative movement, folk, and square dance should be used depending on age and the desired educational outcomes, be they physical, mental, emotional, social, or a combination of any of these results.

A dramatic need in teaching the blind is to build a movement vocabulary. Often verbal meanings need to be established by having the student feel the teacher's movement or be manipulated by the teacher. As sighted teachers, we may have to rethink what we want the children to learn and how to communicate it to children who cannot see. Small classes or assistance from sighted assistants on a near one-to-one basis help children develop movement vocabularies and confidence.

To experience how absence of vision affects movement, wear a blindfold and entrust yourself to a sighted guide. After a time you will develop trust in your partner; then try to leave your partner and move freely in the same space alone. Many blind children — prone to rigid movement — have never experienced the pure delight in running fast. Use of a sighted partner or a safely structured experience can add new dimension to their movement.

Blind children respond better than their sighted equivalents to the use of percussion instruments and rhythmic patterns (Duggar 1968). Quality of movement and sound can stimulate caricatures and dramatic plays, and children can transfer the vibrations of percussive instruments into movement. The adept teacher will find objects or sensations to substitute for the visual learning experiences of other children. But the innate joy of moving freely and imaginatively is no different either for blind or sighted children.

Margaret Duggar and Jo Weisbrod discuss further techniques for working with blind students, and feel the teacher should not further complicate the original handicap through attempting to teach the student formal dances (Duggar *1968*, Weisbrod 1974). Once having helped students to understand movement vocabulary and to be secure in moving through space, the teacher's objectives are the same as for the blind students.

Mental retardation has been, for me, the greatest area of success. My abiding interest in child growth and development helped me to translate the usual chronological descriptions into maturational equivalents and to concentrate on the behavioral evidence of their stage of development. Recently our university hosted "A Very Special Arts Fair" and I was asked to work with dance. I structured a number of movement experiences around action songs, rhythmic instruments, and creative movement. Most traditional action songs, simple circle dances, and creative movement activities can be adapted for use with retarded children once their needs have been analyzed. I asked students from my elementary dance class, as well as a number of music therapy majors to help me throughout the day. Some students verbalized their discomfort with the lack of correlation between the apparent ages of the persons before them and the actual behavioral responses. But many years ago I discovered that the age and behavior of the college students I taught had nothing to do with their dance experience, so I developed a growth and development approach to teaching dance fundamentals. Children walk before they run, jump before they hop, hop before they skip. They learn to stretch and bend before they learn to push and pull, and require both experiences before they strike and dodge. If college students need to learn dance experiences in a logical developmental order, it seemed natural that the retarded child must learn in the same way.

Two areas of work with the handicapped, psychotic and orthopedic, should be the domain of the dance therapist. The dance teacher of the handicapped is meddling here. Both require highly specialized training and knowledge and the lay person can do great damage in spite of good intentions. The same applies to mixed or multiple handicaps as often evidenced in cerebral palsy and muscular dystrophy.

Dance for the Handicapped-New Frontiers?

Dance can be a glorious and integrating experience. History records the use of dance as a religious, therapeutic cure throughout the ages. While we have much to learn, it remains that most humans struggle to unite their beings in a facsimile of human totality. Those with handicaps need others to help them struggle toward that fulfillment. New fields in special education portend fruitful alliances with dance.

Hooray for dance for the handicapped! Enter its doors with praise and thanksgiving that the work of the dance therapists has prepared the way. A saint will learn about the handicapped before attempting to teach them, and a sinner will not care.

References

Duggar, Margaret P. "What Can Dance Be to Someone Who Cannot See?" Washington, D.C.: *Journal of Health, Physical Education and Recreation*, May 1968.

Killilea, Marie. *Karen*, New York: Prentice-Hall, 1952.

Mason, Kathleen C. ed. *Dance Therapy: Focus on Dance VII*. Reston, Virginia: AAHPER, 1974.

Schmais, Claire, "Dance Therapy in Perspective," in *Dance Therapy: Focus on Dance VII*, 4.

Schmais, Claire, "What is Dance Therapy?" *Journal of Health, Phsycial Education and Recreation* January, 1976.

Weisbrod, Jo. "Body Movement Therapy and the Visually-Impaired Person" in *Dance Therapy, Focus on Dance VII, Kathleen Criddle Mason*.

Wisher, Pete, "Therapeutic Values of Dance Education for the Deaf," in *Dance Therapy, Focus on Dance VII*, 1974.

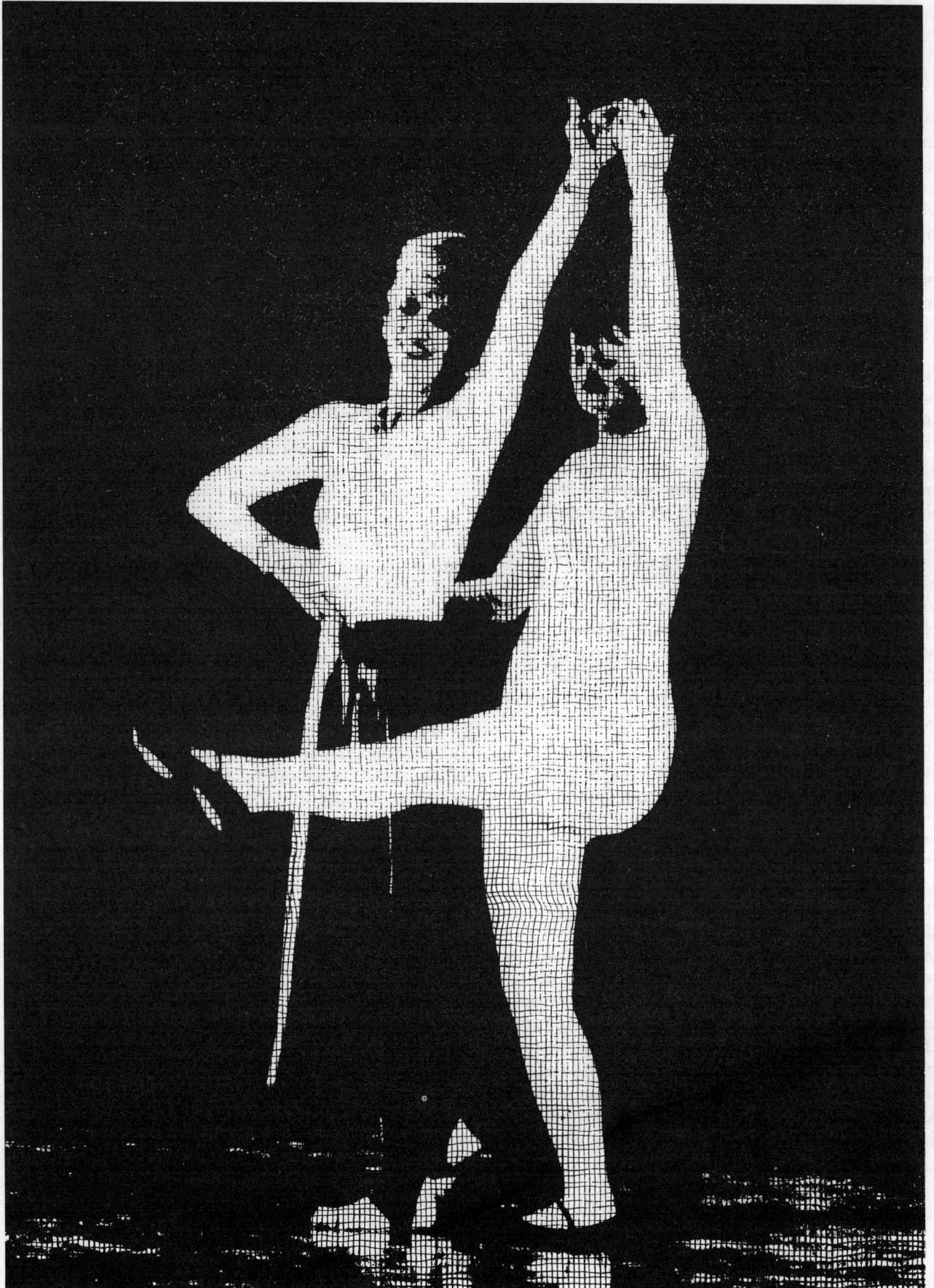

Appendices

⒜ Public Law 94-142 and the Arts*

Claudine Sherrill

Public Law 94-142, the Education for All Handicapped Children Act, was signed by President Gerald Ford on November 29, 1975. Almost two years later, on August 23, 1977, the final rules and regulations for implementing this law were published in the *Federal Register*, Vol. 42, No. 163. Thus a new era began. What are the implications of this law for the arts? What understandings and appreciations must educators and therapists in music, dance, art, and drama have in order to implement the law? This chapter will attempt to answer such questions.

Purpose of the Law

The intent of Congress in passing P.L. 94-142 was to assure quality education for the estimated eight million handicapped children, ages 3-21, in the United States. The following statement comes directly from the law:

> It is the purpose of this Act to assure that all handicapped children have available to them, within the time periods specified, a free appropriate public education which emphasizes special education and related services designed to meet their unique needs (Public Law 94-142, 1975, Sec. 3, c).

Congress conceived of P.L. 94-142 as a Bill of Rights for Handicapped Children. Inherent in this law are four basic rights.

- Right to Free Public Education
- Right to Nondiscriminatory Evaluation
- Right to an Appropriate Education
- Right to Due Process of Law

P.L. 94-142 places responsibility for implementation of the goal of *full educational opportunity* for all handicapped children on the state education agency. In most instances the Special Education Division of the state educational agency will be the driving force behind the goal attainment. It is imperative therefore that arts advocates and/or arts teachers or therapists become knowledgeable about special education, thoroughly conversant with state and local priorities, and personally acquainted with their community's decision-making special educators.

Achieving the Purpose

One way to achieve this task is to join special education professional organizations so that arts advocates are always highly visible at various gatherings. On the other hand, organizations pertaining to arts, music, dance, and drama should invite special educators to participate in their meetings and conferences and should ascertain that key special educators are on their mailing lists. Only by frequent, cooperative sharing of perceptions concerning the meanings of *full educational opportunity* will special educators and arts personnel reach common understandings.

P.L. 94-142, like most legislation, is written in the broadest of terms. Whereas arts advocates may view *full educational opportunity* as including experiences in the arts, others may have entirely different perceptions. Clearly each state education agency, through cooperative planning activities, must develop its own priorities.

Full educational opportunity, as used in P.L. 94-142, simply reflects a civil rights principle. No meaning can be read into the phrase other than the obligation of the public schools to provide free education for all children, ages 3-21, by September 1, 1980 (except in instances where the education of the 3-5 and 18-21 age ranges would be inconsistent with state law or practice or any court decree). P.L. 94-142 mandates that public schools must find ways to meet the educational or training needs of all children regardless of the severity of their handicap. Public schools of the future will have nonambulatory, nonverbal, non-toilet trained children who in the past were considered uneducable. No longer will parents have to pay for special training programs in private or residential schools, nor will they have to provide transportation for severely handicapped children unable to use regular school or city buses. This is the essence of the meaning of full educational opportunity.

*From *Creative Arts for the Severely Handicapped*, 2nd ed., by Claudine Sherrill, 1979. Courtesy of Charles C. Thomas, Publisher, Springfield, Illinois 62717.

References to the Arts in the Rules and Regulations

In developing the official rules and regulations for implementation of P.L. 94-142, two years were devoted to gathering input from all groups which might be affected. Arts advocates, among others, worked arduously to convince decision-makers that specific reference to artistic and cultural activities should appear in the rules and regulations. Success in achieving such reference would lend considerable valence to subsequent cooperative planning of curricula at local levels.

As a result of these efforts, the following direct quotation appears in the comments section of the *Federal Register,* August 23, 1977, following the presentation of *Full Educational Opportunity Goal* (121a. 304).

> *Comment.* In meeting the full educational opportunity goal, the Congress also encouraged local educational agencies to include artistic and cultural activities in programs supported under this part, subject to the priority requirements under 121a.320-121a.324. This point is addressed in the following statements from the Senate Report on Pub. L. 94-142:
>
> The use of the arts as a teaching tool for the handicapped has long been recognized as a viable, effective way not only of teaching special skills, but also of reaching youngsters who had otherwise been unteachable. The Committee envisions that programs under this bill could well include an arts component and, indeed, urges that local educational agencies include arts in programs for the handicapped funded under this Act. Such a program could cover both appreciation of the arts by the handicapped youngsters and the utilization of the arts as a teaching tool per se.

This statement gives arts advocates considerable leverage when interpreting the intent of Congress to local townspeople and soliciting their support in cooperative planning of educational programs for handicapped children. The comment, however, cannot be interpreted as a mandate. It appears only to expand and broaden the awareness of local programmers. Once such awareness exists, tremendous effort is still required to translate it into action.

Another specific mention of the arts appears under *Program Options,* 121a.305, in the *Federal Register,* August 23, 1977. This paragraph reads as follows:

> Each public agency shall take steps to insure that its handicapped children have available to them the variety of educational programs and services available to non-handicapped children in the area served by the agency, including art, music, industrial arts, consumer and homemaking education, and vocational education.

Those school systems which employ art, music, dance, and drama specialist-teachers for instruction within the regular education curriculum must now provide the same variety of program options within special education to be in compliance with the law. Handicapped children must be accorded the right to try out for chorus or band, for a role in the school play, and to submit their original art products in various school contests. Sensitive educators, knowledgeable about the variables which affect self-concept, will insure not only the right to try out but also the right to succeed, at least within the framework of the same normal probability that governs the chance of nonhandicapped children. The law, however, cannot mandate success; this outcome depends entirely upon the value systems and humanistic philosophy of teachers and administrators.

It should be noted that the law does not specify *who* shall provide such program options nor *what* instructional arrangements shall be made available. Nor does it indicate that specially designed and separate arts programs must be developed specifically for the handicapped. In many instances, mainstream arts programs can be expanded to include the handicapped. A new part can be added to the school play or a dance choreography to create a role for a nonverbal or nonambulatory pupil. Musical instruments can be fitted with special adaptations so that physically disabled children can learn to play them. Writing, choreographing, producing, and directing talents can be developed among handicapped children who show creative potential. For pupils who seem to lack both creativity and performance potentials, but who still yearn for involvement, numerous other tasks can be shared: ushering, selling tickets, constructing scenery, moving props, even cooking the traditional after-performance meal.

The Arts in Special Education and in Related Services

The rules and regulations for P.L. 94-142 make only one other specific reference to the arts. To understand it, one must be familiar with the distinction made in the law between *special education* as opposed to *related services.*

Special education is defined as

> . . . specially designed instruction at no cost to parents or guardians, to meet the unique needs of a handicapped child, including classroom instruction, instruction in physical education, home instruction, and instruction in hospitals and institutions. (Sec. 121a.14)

Related services is explained as

> . . . transportation and such developmental, corrective, and other supportive services as are required to assist a handicapped child to benefit from special education, and includes speech pathology and audiology, psychological services, physical and occupational therapy, recreation, early identification and assess-

ment of disabilities in children, counseling services, and medical services for diagnostic and evaluation purposes. The term also includes school health services, social work services in schools, and parent counseling and training. (Sec. 121a.13)

Arts advocates tried hard, but failed to gain a specific reference to the arts within the official definition of related services. They did, however, succeed in achieving a mention within the comments following the definition. Stated verbatim, it says

> *Comment.* With respect to related services, the Senate Report states: . . . the list of related services is not exhaustive and may include other developmental, corrective, or supportive services (such as artistic and cultural programs, and art, music, and dance therapy) if they are required to assist a handicapped child to benefit from special education.

This comment opens the door for the arts as well as their related therapies provided their proponents can convince local educational programmers that such arts services are requisite to a particular child's benefitting from special education. The comment also provokes consideration of the meanings of such words as *developmental, corrective,* and *supportive* which appear to be the determining criteria for inclusion of the arts in the curriculum under the related services provision.

In summary, P.L. 94-142 mandates for all handicapped children *specially designed instruction . . . to* meet their unique needs and *related services* which are required to assist handicapped pupils to benefit from special education. Clearly most handicapped children do not need specially designed instruction in all curricular areas; they can spend some time in the mainstream. Likewise not all handicapped children require related services as defined in the law.

What then determines whether or not a child is receiving an appropriate education? Specifically how can the arts become an integral part of *specially designed instruction* or of *related services?*

The Individualized Educational Program

The right to an appropriate education is guaranteed by P.L. 94-142 by the provision that each handicapped child's specially designed instruction shall evolve from an *individualized education program* (IEP) written specifically for him. A meeting must be held at least once a year for the specific purpose of reviewing this IEP and, if appropriate, revising its provisions. The public agency must insure that this meeting includes the child's teacher, one other school representative who is knowledgeable about special education, one or both parents, the child when appropriate, and other individuals at the discretion of the parent or agency.

The right to appropriate education then is protected by cooperative planning and review of the handicapped child's specially designed instruction and requisite related services. P.L. 94-142 specifies the content which the resulting IEP must include:

a) A statement of the child's present levels of educational performance;
b) A statement of annual goals, including short term instructional objectives;
c) A statement of the specific special education and related services to be provided to the child, and the extent to which the child will be able to participate in regular educational programs;
d) The projected dates for initiation of services and the anticipated duration of the services; and
e) Appropriate objective criteria and evaluation procedures and schedules for determining, on at least an annual basis, whether the short term instructional objectives are being achieved (Sec. 121a.346).

The extent to which the arts appear within the components of the individualized educational program entirely depends upon the participants in the cooperative planning and review process. Teachers and parents aware of the values of the arts for their own sake and/or as lead up activities or teaching tools may infiltrate the IEP with specific short term instructional objectives in the arts. They may write in specially designed arts instruction to meet unique needs and/or they may specify a certain percentage of time each day or week in mainstream arts instruction. In the case of a nonverbal autistic child, they may write in the related services of a dance, music, or art therapist. In the case of a teenager with severe socialization deficits which prevent academic learning, they may write in the related services of a recreation specialist skilled in the use of the arts to facilitate improved social skills.

The potential within the IEP for prescribing the arts as content and/or as process is subject to only the boundaries of human vision. Full realization of such possibilities rests with school systems in which arts specialists, parents, and special educators have learned and shared together for many years. Much caring, trusting, and compromising occur in cooperative planning endeavors leading to some of the new integrated arts approaches to learning. Territorial hostilities among the separate disciplines of art, music, dance, and drama must disappear. The dichotomy between education and therapy must be resolved.

Preservice and Inservice Training Needs

The old adage, a journey of a thousand miles begins with a single step, seems appropriate. If the arts are to become an integral part of the education of hand-icapped children, preservice and inservice training of teachers and paraprofessionals must be drastically changed. Special educators must be expected to develop understandings, appreciations, and skills in the arts and the creative process.

Arts educators and/or therapists must achieve competencies in evaluation and assessment, in describing present levels of educational performance, in writing short term instructional objectives, in teaching handicapped children in the mainstream and a variety of other instructional arrangements, and in evaluating the behavioral changes which occur in handicapped children as a result of participation in the arts and the creative process.

The many tasks involved in direct service delivery within the arts can be organized under three broad areas as depicted in Chart 1: Learner Assessment and Counseling, Program Implementation and Evaluation, and Artist-Educator Community Leadership. These roles, whether actualized by educators, artists, recreators, or parents, can be adapted to the home or residential facility, the school, or the creative arts facilities in the community.

Following the chart is an illustrative taxonomy of tasks associated with the three broad role areas. These tasks can serve as the basis for developing learning modules for inclusion in inservice education workshops and leadership institutes.

Chart 1. Personnel Roles in Creative Arts Education for the Handicapped

LEARNER ASSESSMENT PLANNING	PROGRAM IMPLEMENTATION AND EVALUATION				COMMUNITY LEADERSHIP
Assessment of present level of creative arts performance: Participating Discovering Feeling Sharing Shaping	**SCHOOL**				Identification and use of arts resource
	Mainstream Regular education setting or least restrictive environment		**Resource Room** Individual instruction Small group instruction		Advocacy
	COMMUNITY				Elimination of barriers
	Mainstream Regular		**Special Resource**		
	Attending performances	Participating in creative arts	Attending performances given especially for handicapped	Participating in activities especially for handicapped	Legislation
Assessment of present level of creative arts appreciations					Litigation
					Consumer involvement
	HOME				
Assessment of leisure time preferences and practices	Family creative arts activities in which handicapped child participates		Individual creative arts endeavors by handicapped person alone or one supportive family or friend		Employment of handicapped
					Action research
Leisure counseling Individual Family Significant others					
IEP Tasks					

Taxonomy of Tasks Associated with Personnel Roles in Creative Arts Education for Handicapped Children and Youth

Tasks Associated with the Role of Assessment and Counseling

1.1 Uses effective procedures for collecting information about present level of creative arts performance, leisure preferences, and practices of each student (client) and his family members.

    1.11 Makes effective use of informal procedures: oral questionnaires, preferences and practice inventories, and interviews on video and audio tapes; anecdotal records; pictorial checklists.

    1.12 Uses standardized test data when appropriate for severely handicapped.

    1.13 Constructs new instruments or modifies and/or adapts ones to performance levels of severely handicapped.

1.2 Uses the appropriate leisure counseling orientation and extends existing identifiable models to include and/or focus on the creative arts.

    1.21 Adapts avocational, recreation, and activities models to severely handicapped.

    1.22 Adapts developmental-educational models to severely handicapped.

    1.23 Adapts normalization models to severely handicapped.

1.3 Assists student (client) and significant others (including family members) in understanding and appreciating self and creative arts potential.

    1.31 Cooperatively explores potential for participating, discovering, feeling, sharing, and shaping ideas in creative/expressive arts.

    1.32 Cooperatively explores potential for attending, observing, enjoying, appreciating, understanding, and criticizing art performances and products of others.

1.4 Works effectively with specialized services and resources.

    1.41 Encourages community recreation personnel to identify and share resources for creative arts education.

    1.42 Encourages civic organizations to help with transportation, cost, volunteer instruction, etc.

    1.43 Encourages artistic and administrative directors of museums, studios, and other facilities to extend services to handicapped.

1.5 Uses IEP (Individualized Educational Planning) model as described in P.L. 94-142 to structure creative arts assessment and planning into a viable instructional program.

    1.51 Includes in IEP a statement of present levels of creative arts performance.

    1.52 Includes in IEP a statement of annual goals for creative arts education and leisure time use, including short term specific behavioral objectives.

    1.53 Includes in IEP a statement of the creative arts services to be provided.

    1.54 Includes in IEP the projected date for initiation of creative arts services and anticipated duration of such services.

    1.55 Includes in IEP evaluation procedures for determining discrepancy between objectives and actual performance after set periods of purposive intervention (instructional, recreational, therapeutic).

Tasks Associated with the Role of Program Implementation and Evaluation

2.1 Adapts principles of growth and development to planning of creative arts activities.

    2.11 Recognizes psychomotor prerequisites to creative arts participation: head and neck control, sufficient muscle tonus; grasp and release mechanisms; fine muscle coordination.

    2.12 Adapts creative arts materials and media accordingly.

2.2 Plans teaching-learning creative arts situations in accordance with acceptable principles of learning.

    2.21 Provides for effective and continuing motivation.

    2.22 Uses a variety of learning experiences broken down according to level of difficulty.

    2.23 Helps student (client) make application of his learning experiences to varied leisure settings at home and in the community.

2.3 Demonstrates professional level in instructional competence.

    2.31 Provides evidence that instruction changes student's level of creative arts performance.

    2.32 Provides evidence that learning experiences increase breadth and/or depth of leisure preferences.

    2.33 Provides evidence that learning experiences change leisure time practices in a positive manner.

2.4 Provides physical environment that facilitates creative arts learning.

    2.41 Adapts musical instruments, arts and crafts equipment and supplies, and other creative arts media and materials to special needs of learner.

    2.42 Controls heat, light, ventilation.

2.43 Provides adequate structure and eliminates irrelevant stimuli.

2.44 Eliminates architectural barriers.

2.5 Evaluates continuously as an integral part of instructional process.

2.51 Involves students and significant others in evaluation of self, teacher, and program.

2.52 Uses resulting data to improve creative arts learning experiences.

2.6 Uses community resources to enhance and reinforce creative arts learnings.

2.61 Uses handicapped adults in the community as role models and artist-educators.

2.62 Takes advantage of creative arts expertise of volunteers in the community.

2.63 Solicits help from professional organizations like National Association of Retarded Citizens and civic organizations like Jaycees.

2.64 Ascertains that students have direct access to all creative arts resources in community.

2.65 Develops in students responsibility for caring for and protecting art products found in the community.

2.66 Helps students to acquire value systems which cherish and protect the arts as an essential right of all American citizens.

Tasks Associated with the Role of Leadership in the Community

3.1 Participates in the definition and solution of community problems relating to creative arts for the handicapped.

3.2 Interprets to others legislation, and possible litigation, which protects rights of the handicapped.

3.3 Acts as an advocate for the severely handicapped and works for extension of their educational-vocational-leisure opportunities to include increasing amounts of the creative arts.

3.4 Works closely with the press and other media in presenting and interpreting the educational and leisure needs and potentials of the severely handicapped to the public.

3.5 Initiates and carries through research pertaining to discrepancies between creative arts education and services received by handicapped vs nonhandicapped populations; pertaining to behavioral changes in handicapped after exposure to creative arts education; pertaining to attitudinal changes of selected groups concerning creative arts potential and performance of the severely handicapped; etc.

Andrews, Gladys, *Creative Rhythmic Movement for Children*. Englewood Cliffs, New Jersey: Prentice-Hall, Inc., 1954.
Explores movement in relation to child development and creativity. Sections cover: movement exploration, development of movement, effects of space and rhythm on movement, making percussion instruments, ideas and compositions for movement, and music and progressions for dance.

Barlin, Anne, and Barlin, Paul. *The Art of Learning Through Movement*. Los Angeles, California: The Ward Ritchie Press, 1971.
Teachers' manual of movement for students of all ages. Representative of chapters: Involvement Through Stories; Involvement Through Fantasy; Vigorous Movement; Moving with Others; Involvement Through Games; Movement Isolations; Involvement Through Dramatic Play; Involvement Through Emotional Expression; Moving Through Space; and Using Movement in Other Classroom Subjects. General hints and first lesson plans are included.

Blankenburg, W. "Tanz in der Therapie Schizophrener (Dance in the Therapy of Schizophrenics)." *Psychotherapy and Psychosomatics* 17: 5-6, 336-342; 1962.
Describes the use of dance as a therapeutic modality in the treatment of schizophrenia. Various dances from different epochs in the history of dance are employed.

Calder, Jean E. "Dance for the Mentally Retarded." *Slow Learning Child* 19:2: 67-78, July 1972.
The role of dance in education and particularly in the education of the mentally retarded is discussed. Considered are dance programs, class size, selection of types of dances, the variety of accompaniments possible, and the role of the teacher. A review of research relating to the place of dance in programs for the mentally retarded and to the significance of dance program in perceptual-motor development programs is presented.

Canner, Norma. *. . . and a Time to Dance*. Boston, Massachusetts: Beacon Press, 1968.
The use of creative movement and dance to help young retarded children is described through narrative and 125 photographs representing the physical and emotional growth of a class through activities and techniques. Teaching methods are suggested for circle activities, nonparticipants, isolation of body parts, locomotor movements, activities with sound, instruments, and rest period objectives and procedures. A discussion of teachers' workshops is included.

Carroccio, Dennis P., and Quattlehaum, Lawrence F. "An Elementary Technique for Manipulation of Participation in Ward Dances at a Neuropsychiatric Hospital." *Journal of Music Therapy* 6:4: 108-109; 1969.
Discusses ways to increase participation in a weekly dance through manipulation of environmental variables.

Chadwick, Ida F. "Historical Aspects of Dance Therapy." *Journal of Physical Education and Recreation* 48:1: 46,48; January 1977.
Author traces the historical philosophies of dance as therapy.

Chapman, Ann, and Cramer, Miriam. *Dance and the Blind Child*. New York, New York: American Dance Guild, Inc. (1619 Broadway, Room 203, 10019), 1973.
Details teaching one blind child in a class of sighted children. Includes eight pages of lesson plans.

---

[1]The bulk of these references are taken from *Materials on Creative Arts (Arts, Crafts, Dance, Drama, Music and Biliotherapy)* for *Persons with Handicapping Conditions*, a project of the Information and Research Utilization Center (IRUC) of AAHPERD. Additional entries are taken from a "Selected Bibliography for Dance for the Handicapped, 1978" a project of the National Committee, Arts for the Handicapped (Suite 801, 1701 K Street, N.W., Washington, D.C. 20006) and AAHPERD.

Cherry, Clare. *Creative Movement for the Developing Child: A Nursery School Handbook for Non-Musicans*. Belmont, California: Fearon Publishers (Education Division of Lear Siegler, Inc.), 1968.

Includes activities to develop more acute sensory perception through movement during different stages of children's growth. Songs, chants, activities, and games foster skills development in crawling, creeping, walking, running, jumping, skipping, whole body movements, kinesthetic awareness, throwing and catching, balance, space orientation, hand movement, and other sensory-motor and perceptual skills.

Costonis, Maureen N. *Therapy in Motion*. Urbana, Illinois: University of Illinois Press, 1978.

Lists about 400 sources of information for dance and therapy for persons with handicapping conditions.

Duggar, Margaret P. "What Can Dance Be to Someone Who Cannot See?" *Journal of Health, Physical Education and Recreation* 39:5: 28-30; May 1968.

Methods for teaching blind children to dance are suggested, including establishing a verbal vocabulary of movement and using analogies and images. Also explained are methods of developing spatial awareness, body awareness, and rhythmic perception, and of using instruments for matching quality of sound and motion.

Fait, Hollis F. *Special Physical Education, Adapted, Corrective, Developmental*. Philadelphia, Pennsylvania: W. B. Saunders Company, 1966.

Written for prospective physical education teachers in a variety of settings. Discusses visual handicaps, auditory handicaps, cerebral palsy, orthopedic defects, heart conditions, convalescence, nutritional disturbances, other physical conditions requiring adapted physical education: mental retardation, social maladjustment, mental illness, and aging. The following activities and topics are treated: basic skill games, rhythms and dance, individual sports, dual games, team games, swimming, weight training, outdoor education, corrective body mechanics, and developmental programs for physical fitness. An appendix includes suggested films and filmstrips for teachers, film sources, record sources, professional societies and associations, and periodicals.

Farina, Albert M., and others. *Growth Through Play*. Englewood Cliffs, New Jersey: Prentice-Hall, Inc., 1959.

Planned to supply a single source for play activities, songs, games, and dances appropriate to ages four through twelve. Helpful to teachers, parents, recreation leaders.

Gewertz, Joanna. "Dance for Psychotic Children." *Journal of Health, Physical Education, and Recreation* 35:1: 63-64; January 1964.

Describes the sessions of a dance therapy program for fifteen psychotic children. Discusses methods to elicit participation. Program led by a volunteer teacher.

Glass. Henry "Buzz". *Action Time – With Story, Chant, and Rhyme (Vol. I)*. Hayward, California: Alameda County School Department (244 West Winton Avenue, 94544), 1973.

Collection of 256 chants and rhymes intended to involve the child with the word in action through dramatics, verse choir, chant, rhyme, story, music, and movement exploration. Subject matter ranges from rocks, spacemen, rain, clouds, vines, flowers, cowboys, warriors, baseball, football, fishing, boats, and storms, and many animal activities.

Grassman, Cyrus S. "Modified Folk and Square Dancing for the Mentally Retarded." *The Physical Educator* 15:1: 32-35; March 1958.

Provides modifications for four standard dances which can be used with groups of mentally retarded age 7-12, IQ 50-75. Includes record needed, formation, movement per measure, words when used, and other possible adaptations. Dances include "Bingo," "Seven Steps," "Masquerade," and "Waltz Quadrille."

Hecox, Bernadette; Levine, Ellen; and Scott, Diana. "A Report on the Use of Dance in Physical Rehabilitation: Every Body has a Right to Feel Good." *Rehabilitation Literature* 36:1: 11-16; January 1975.

Describes and evaluates a dance program for physically handicapped adults at St. Luke's Hospital, New York City. Five case studies illustrate values of dance.

Hill, Kathleen. *Dance for Physically Disabled Persons: A Manual for Teaching Ballroom, Square, and Folk Dances to Users of Wheelchairs and Crutches*. Washington, D. C.: American Alliance for Health, Physical Education, and Recreation, June 1976.

Huberty, C. J.; Quirk, J. P.; and Swan, W. "Dance Therapy with Psychotic Children." *Archives of General Psychiatry* 28:5: 707-713; May 1973.

The development and evaluation of a dance program are described. The program, designed to modify a variety of irregular and disordered body-movement patterns common to psychotic children, was conducted in a day-care unit.

King, Bruce. *Creative Dance: Experience for Learning.* Blawenburg, New Jersey: Dance World Books, 1968.
Introduces creative dance teaching for children. Discusses: creative dance in elementary education, principles and techniques of creative teaching, and children's interests that can be used for dance. One section deals with the teacher's skills and attitude. A bibliography is included.

Kratz, L. E. *Movement Without Sight.* Palo Alto, California: Peek Publications, 1973.
Provides a definition of blindness, the role of relaxation, and posture and locomotion. Activities cover individual stunts and self-testing, rhythms, and dance.

Kraus, Richard. *Pocket Guide of Folk and Square Dances and Singing Games.* Englewood Cliffs, New Jersey: Prentice Hall, Inc., 1966.
This book is designed for elementary grades, but it could be used in some instances with older mentally retarded individuals. Includes such activities as "Five Little Chickadees," "Mulberry Bush," "Virginia Reel," "Maypole Dance," "Salty Dog Rag," and square dancing.

Kubitsky-Kaltman. *Teachers' Dance Handbook No. 1.* Freeport, New York: Educational Activities, Inc. (P. O. Box 392, 11520), n.d.
Outlines a program progression based on growth and development. Begins with rhymes, songs, plays, and simple dances to more advanced national dances of many countries. Explicit directions and tunes are included in each dance.

Latchaw, and Pyatt. *A Pocket Guide of Dance Activities.* Englewood Cliffs, New Jersey: Prentice Hall, Inc., 1958.
Gives explicit directions for movement experiences in play acting, creative movement, music with movement, gradually working from simple nursery rhyme dances to popular folk dances.

Mason, Kathleen Criddle, ed. *Dance Therapy: Focus on Dance VII.* Reston, VA: American Alliance for Health, Physical Education, and Recreation, 1974.
Compilation of articles exploring the development, theory, and methods of dance therapy. Philosophy and methods are examined for the dance therapist in a psychiatric setting, as a member of a clinical team, in group therapy, and in individual work. Techniques for research and observation are examined. Dance is discussed for the following special groups: children with minimal brain dysfunction, the visually-impaired, the deaf, children with emotional or learning problems, and older people. Training and professional status is examined and a dance therapy consultant model presented.

Matteson, Carol A. "Finding the Self in Space." *Music Educators Journal* 58:8: 63-65, 135; April 1972.
Use of motor development activities, physical activities, and music with handicapped children is discussed. Use of movement and spatial relationship in music classes with multiply handicapped children is advocated to aid growth of body and mind. Practical guidelines for children with various handicaps to learn about the qualities of movement and sound are presented.

Moran-Kalakian. *Movement Experiences for the Mentally Retarded or Emotionally Disturbed Child.* Minneapolis: Burgess Publishing Co., 1977.

Mossman, Maja. "Movement — The Joyous Language: Dance Therapy for Children." *Children's House* 8:5: 11-15; Spring 1976.

Nagel, Charles, and Moore, Fredricka. *Skill Development Through Games and Rhythmic Activities.* Palo Alto, California: The National Press, 1966.
Material presented is useful to personnel directing skill development for various age groups. Skills are related to practice in these areas: goals and purposes for developing movement skills; ball skills; rhythm skills; advanced ball skills; team games; dance skills for folk and social dance. The carefully worked out progressions and many sequential illustrations make the contents appropriate for those who work with the mentally retarded in physical education or recreation programs.

National Dance Association *Guidelines for Children's Dance.* Reston, VA: American Alliance for Health, Physical Education, and Recreation, 1971.
Based on a 1969 survey of elementary physical education programs, discusses the status of dance and the professional preparation of those responsible for dance instruction in the elementary school Defines objectives, general approach, and methods for dance instruction. Provides guidelines for movement-centered activities central to the dance curriculum from early through middle childhood.

Paley, A. M. "Dance Therapy: An Overview" *American Journal of Psychoanalysis* 34: 81-83; 1974.

Perlumutter, Ruth. "Dance Me a Cloud." *Children's House* 6:6: 15-19; Winter 1974.
Describes how a dance-movement program for inner-city children uses creative dance to help children communicate with their bodies what they cannot through language. Several techniques which promote free expression are explained in-

cluding: the "magic circle" exercises to explore and express emotions; space; space as a shape; touch; the importance of touch; and activities which serve to release tension.

Polk, Elizabeth. "Notes on the Demonstration of Dance Technique and Creative Dance as Taught to Deaf Children, Ages 7-11." *Journal of the American Dance Therapy Association, Inc.* 1:1: 4-5; Fall 1968.
Methods and techniques for teaching deaf children to dance.

Recreation Literature Retrieval Project. "Selected Bibliography on Recreation for the Mentally Retarded." *Therapeutic Recreation Journal* 3:4: 14, 41-42; 1968.
A bibliography of 34 selected items, covering materials published between April 1964 and July 1968. Activities include crafts, games, dance, scouting, and camping. Other areas of concern are motor function improvement, social education, cultural deprivation, model cities, adolescent attitudes, home influences, activities programing, and physical education. A project of the Recreation and Parks Program, the Pennsylvania State University, College Park, Pennsylvania.

Robbins, Ferris, and Robbins, Jennet. *Educational Rhythmics for Mentally and Physically Handicapped Children.* New York, New York: Association Press, 1968.
Presents the use of foundational rhythmic and movement skills correlated to the participants education program. Detailed progression of activities are well illustrated and easily understood.

Robbins, Ferris, and Robbins, Jannet. *Supplement to Educational Rhythmics for Mentally and Physically Handicapped Children.* Zurich, Switzerland: Ra-Verlag, Rapperswil, 1966.
This supplement is a continuation of original book *Educational Rhythmics for Mentally Handicapped Children.* Motor action and coordinated movement, accompanied by music, the spoken word, vision, touch, and the natural sense of imitation are discussed.

————. *Educational Rhythmics for Mentally Handicapped Children.* New York: Horizon Press, 1965.
Using fundamental rhythms with the retarded, program utilizes music, words, pictures, and movements to achieve total child development. Exercises are given for the severely retarded, intermediate, and more advanced.

Roberts, A. G. "Dance Movement Therapy: Adjunctive Treatment in Psychotherapy." *Canada's Mental Health* 22:4: 11; December 1974.

Robinson, Christopher, and others. *Physical Activity in the Education of Slow-Learning Children.* Baltimore, Maryland: Williams and Wilkins Co., 1970.
Guide to physical activity for mentally handicapped children. Activities, materials and teaching methods are recommended for nursery through adolescent age groups in four main areas: educational gymnastics (to learn functional body management), educational dance (to learn to move expressively), skills and games (to learn handing of balls, bats, etc., to be able to participate in games and sports), and specific posture training, which includes corrective exercises for simple muscular or postural defects.

Robinson, Violeta Compagnoni. *The Effects of Psycho-dance with Neuro-Psychiatric Patients.* Master's thesis. Jacksonville, Illinois: MacMurry College, 1957.

Rosen, Elizabeth Ruth. *Dance in the Therapy of Psychotic Patients.* Doctoral dissertation. New York: Columbia University, 1956.

Samoore, Rhoda. "A Rhythm Program for Hearing Impaired Children." *The Illinois Advance.* 1-3, 15-20; January 1970.
A rhythm program based on the conviction that teaching rhythmic bodily movements and an appreciation of music facilitate speech development in deaf students at both the primary and secondary level. Benefits are cited and objectives outlined for oral and manual rhythm programs. The methods and content of the rhythm classes are detailed (body and voice exercises, auditory discrimination practice, examples of songs and dances, vocabulary development and speech practice techniques, and development of an appreciation and knowledge of musical instruments).

Sandel, Susan L. "Integrating Dance Therapy into Treatment." *Hospital and Community Psychiatry* 26:7: 439-440; July 1975.

Schmais, Claire. "What is Dance Therapy." *Journal of Physical Education and Recreation* 47:1: 39; January 1976.
Explores differences between dance therapy and teaching. Although good dance teaching is therapeutic, dance as therapy requires intentional therapeutic intervention.

————. "What Dance Therapy Teaches Us About Teaching Dance." *Journal of Health, Physical Education, and Recreation* 41:1: 34-35, 88; January 1970.
The underlying purpose of dance therapy, reinforcing the ability to communicate, is reflected through

experiences and comments of a dance therapist. Attention is given to important elements of a dance session and the use of effort-shape theory to give meaning to movement. Explores the structure of a typical dance class, the growth of social interaction as a result, using dances from other countries to express other people's culture and modern dance in relation to dance therapy.

Schniderman, Craig M., and Volkman, Ann. "Music and Movement Involve the Whole Child." *Teaching Exceptional Children* 7:2: 58-60; Winter 1975.
Camp Greentree (Bethesda, Maryland) is a therapeutic day camp for emotionally disturbed boys. Music and movement experiences are provided to alleviate psychological stress of disturbed, aggressive children.

Szyman, Robert. "Square Dancing on Wheels." *Sports 'n Spokes* 2:4: 5-7; November-December 1976.
Nearly 50 persons are members of the Colorado Wheelers, a square dance club for individuals in wheelchairs. How to form such a club, as well as basic square dance maneuvers, are discussed in this article.

Thieler, Virginia L. *A Study of Behavior in a Boys' Dance Therapy Group at St. Elizabeth's Hospital.* Unpublished master's thesis. Washington, D. C.: Catholic University of America, 1950.

Tipple, Blanche. "Dance Therapy and Education Program." *Journal of Leisurability* 2:4: 9-12; October 1975.
Describes the dance therapy program at Muskoka Centre (Gravenhurst, Ontario). Over 150 mentally retarded residents participate in ballet, tap, acrobatics, and ballroom dancing.

Weisbrod, Jo Anne. "Shaping a Body Image Through Movement Therapy." *Music Educators Journal* 58:8: 66-69; April 1972.

Wisher, Peter R. "Dance and the Deaf." *Journal of Health, Physical Education, and Recreation* 40:3: 81; 1969.
Discusses considerations for hearing impaired participants in dance activities. Accompaniment, tactile cues, creativity, balance, relationship to speech development, student interest, and program values are covered.

Witkin, Kate. *To Move, To Learn.* Philadelphia: Temple University Press, 1977.

ⓒ Contributors

Gertrude Blanchard
15 Jessen Court
Kensington, CA 94707

Dan Cieloha
1422 Oxford Street
Berkeley, CA 94709

Faith Clark, Ph.D.
Department of Physical Education
Western Illinois University
Macomb, IL 61455

Cynthia Crain, M.A.
Division of Health, Physical Education, and
    Recreation
Virginia Polytechnic Institute and State University
Blacksburg, VA 24061

Sally Fitt, Ed.D.
Modern Dance Department
University of Utah
Salt Lake City, UT 84112

Carol Kay Harsell, M.A.
Dance and Motor Development Consultant
8310 East McDonald, 3104
Scottsdale, AZ 85253

Madeline Hunter, Ed.D.
University Elementary School
University of California at Los Angeles
Los Angeles, CA 90024

Marcia Leventhal, M.A., D.T.R.
Director, Graduate Dance Therapy Program
    Department of Dance and Dance Education
New York University
New York, NY 10012

Marcia L. Lloyd
Department of Physical Education
Idaho State University
Pocatello, Idaho 83209

Kathleen C. Mason, M.Ed., D.T.R.
Department of Special Education
Granite School District
Salt Lake City, UT 84109

Aida Pisciotta, M.F.A.
Department of Physical Education
Iowa State University
Ames, IA 50010

Rebecca Reber, M.A.
1824 Concord Lane
Denton, TX 76201

Anne Riordan
Modern Dance Department/Special Education
University of Utah
Salt Lake City, UT 84112

Nancy Brooks Schmitz, M.F.A.
Department of Drama/Dance
University of Montana
Missoula, MT 59801

Claudine Sherrill, Ed.D.
Department of Physical Education
Texas Woman's University
Denton, TX 76204

Julian Stein, Ed.D.
Information and Research Utilization Center in
    Physical Education and Recreation for the
    Handicapped
American Alliance for Health, Physical Education,
    Recreation and Dance
Reston, VA 22091

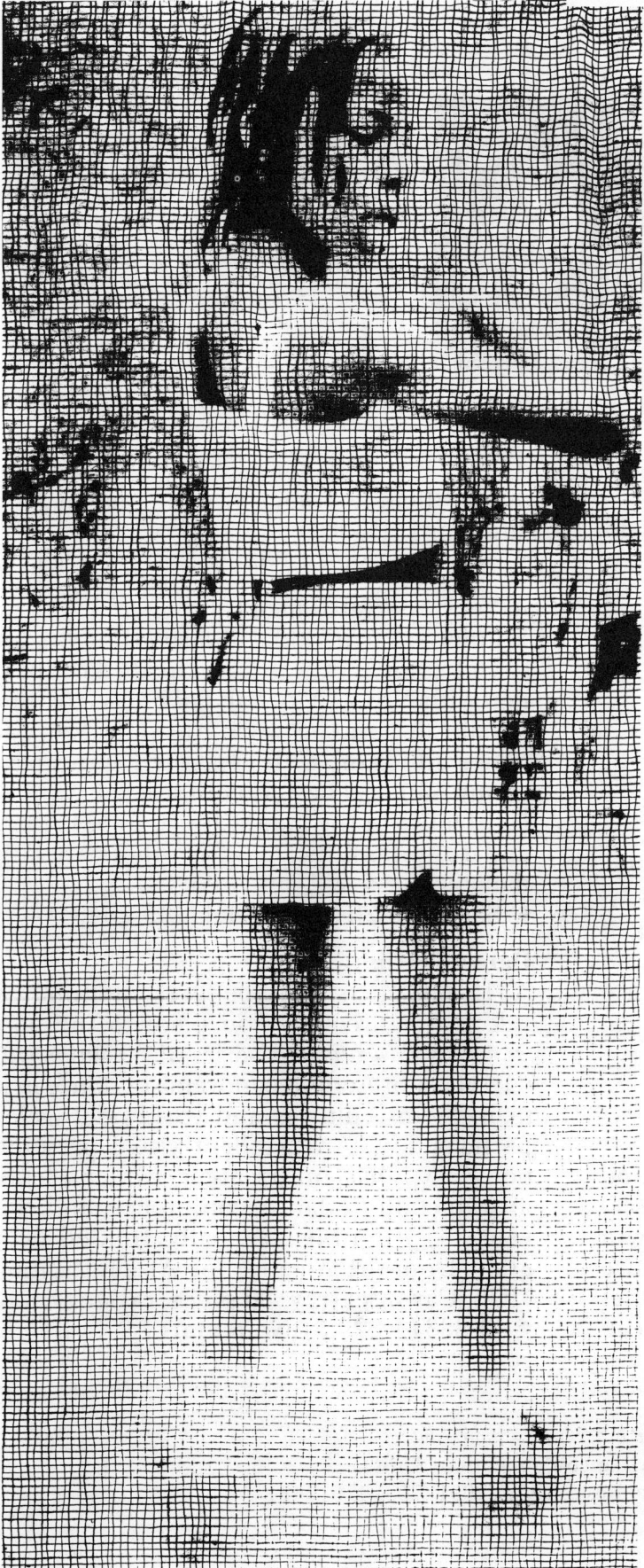

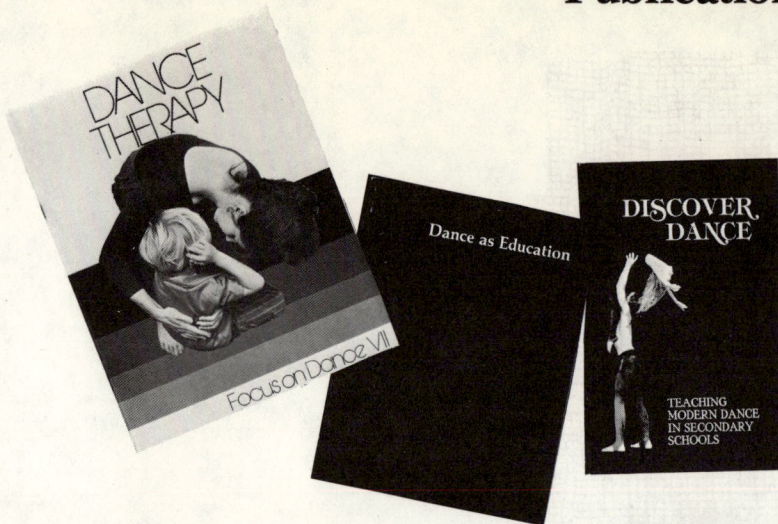

Focus on Dance VII—Dance Therapy

A comprehensive examination of the field. Articles on training, research, methods of work, and dance therapy for special groups by leaders in one of dance's most exciting fields. 1974.

- 80 pp. (0-88314-072-1)

Dance as Education

A position paper providing information essential for creating, guiding, evaluating, and defending dance experiences in the schools. Topics focus on issues and concerns in dance education such as: the what and why of dance, dance in education and the right of access to dance, curricula in dance, and teachers and specialists in dance. Contains a widely-endorsed resolution on dance education. 1977.

- 56 pp. (0-88314-051-9)

Discover Dance

Presents basic ideas, potential values, and suggested activities for teachers on the secondary level. Provides administrators with the basic framework for developing a dance curriculum. Ideas, activities, and guidelines are presented in such a way that teachers can adapt them to their own unique teaching situations. 1978.

- 80 pp. (0-88314-060-8)

A Very Special Dance (film)

Winner of 5 national awards, this 16 mm sound color film was developed in cooperation with NBC/TV of Salt Lake City, focusing specifically on the work of Anne Riordan, dance educator, with mentally handicapped young adults. The audience sees the wonderful abilities of the handicapped to be creative and to communicate with others through dance.

- Sale (243-26402) Rental (243-26404)

Dance Is (film)

A 12-minute slide-tape presentation, developed as a companion piece to the book *Dance As Education*. A series of 80 slides with narration presents a panorama of dance in its many forms, cultures, and worldwide, ageless participation. An excellent visual presentation for public information, career classes, introduction to dance, conference, and convention programs. Partially funded by a grant from the Alliance for Arts Education. 1978. Carousel tray, 80 slides, cassette.

- (0-88314-229-5) **No rentals**

For price and order information, contact
American Alliance Publications Unit
1900 Association Drive, Reston, VA 22091 (703) 476–3481